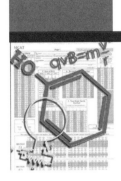

MCAT:
THE ANSWER KEY

...In Plain English

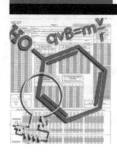

Other Books from Indus Publishing Corporation

The Complete Guide to Foreign Medical Schools:
In Plain English

Control Yourself!

The Non-Trivial Trivia Book

SAT I :The Answer Key
In Plain English

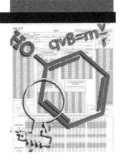

MCAT:
THE ANSWER KEY

In Plain English

by

Nilanjan Sen

Indus Publishing Corporation

Wayland · New York

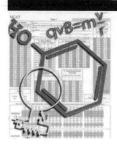

Indus Publishing Corporation
7052 Pokey Moonshine
Wayland, NY 14572
Fax: 716-728-9756
E-mail: induspub@aol.com

ISBN: 1-890838-05-5
Library of Congress: 98-75475

Credits:

Editing: Frank Mochol
         Dr. David Meisel
         Christopher Werth
         Laura Cancilla

Cover Design: Linda Ann Scura

Manufactured in the United States of America

AUTHOR

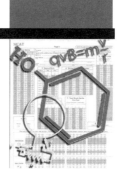

Nilanjan Sen is an honors graduate of the University of Rochester (BA) and New York University Graduate School (MA). Mr. Sen has many years of research experience in the field of medical sciences. He has served as an Assistant Professor of Biology at Westchester Community College. Over the years Mr. Sen has been associated with the nation's leading test-preparation companies, currently serving as Chairman of Test Prep International, a worldwide leader in test preparation services. In addition to his business ventures, Sen is an accomplished science writer. He serves as the Chairman and the primary science writer for Indus Publishing Corporation. Other books written by Mr. Sen include: Genetics Review - Cliffs Notes (1997), Cracking the Chemistry Regents Examination - The Princeton Review - Random House (1998), Chemistry Review - The Princeton Review - Random House (1998), The Complete Guide To Foreign Medical Schools - Indus Publishing Corporation (1997), The Non-Trivial Trivia Book - Indus Publishing Corporation (1997).

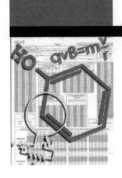

CONTENT BY SECTIONS

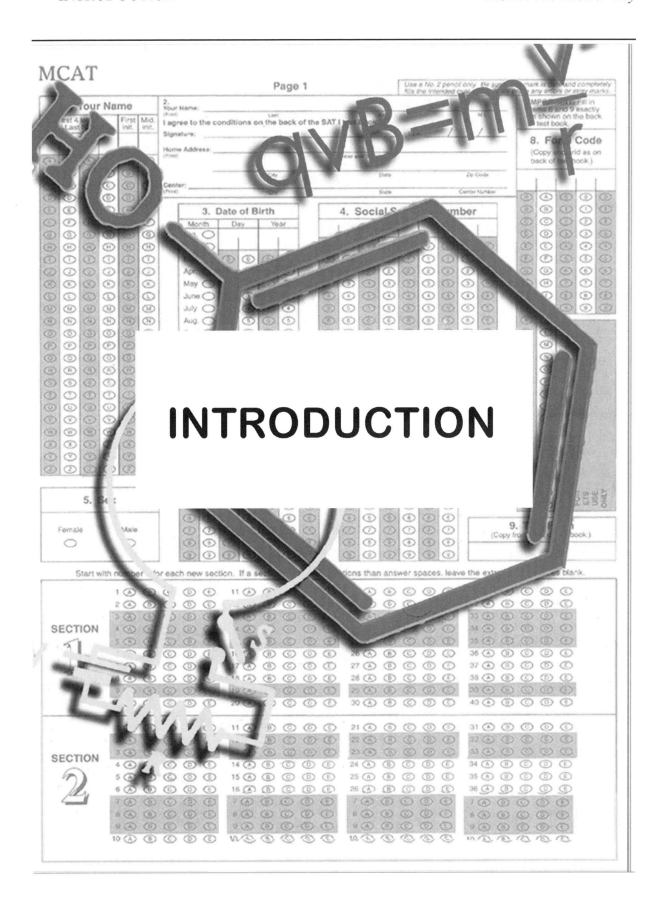

INTRODUCTION

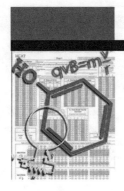

INTRODUCTION

The MCAT: The Answer Key aims to help students approach their goals realistically. The book contains information that a student needs to know in pithy manner. Why waste time with books that are encyclopedic in nature, when you can study the facts that you need to know by using ready-to-go index cards? Just tear out the perforated cards and start studying.

Medical school admission requirements vary from school to school. Each school's specific prerequisites are detailed in the Medical School Admission Requirements (MSAR), an annual   publication of the Association of American Medical Colleges (AAMC). The MSAR is highly recommended to all prospective applicants and is available at most school libraries and premedical advising offices.

In general, most medical schools will expect applicants to have attempted the Medical College Admission Test (MCAT), and to have completed the following types of courses:

One year of BIOLOGY
One year of PHYSICS
One year of ENGLISH
Two years of CHEMISTRY (through Organic Chemistry)

Applicants should also consider volunteering at a local hospital or clinic to gain practical experience in the health professions. In addition, a well-rounded sample of extra-curricular activities or work experiences, both related and unrelated to medicine, will help broaden an applicant's knowledge and development.

The Medical College Admission Test (MCAT) is a standardized, multiple-choice examination designed to assist admission committees in predicting which of their applicants will perform adequately in the medical school curriculum. The test assesses problem solving, critical thinking, and writing skills in addition to the examinee's knowledge of science concepts and principles prerequisite to the study of medicine. The MCAT is scored in each of the following areas: Verbal Reasoning, Physical Sciences, Writing Sample, and Biological Sciences.

Nearly all U.S. medical schools require applicants to attempt the MCAT before applying for admission. Please note that the format of the MCAT changed with the 1991 administration. Most schools will require applicants to take the new test and will not accept older scores. Applicants should refer to the Medical School Admission Requirements (MSAR) to determine specific MCAT requirements.

Registration for the MCAT may be obtained by contacting: MCAT Program Office P.O. Box 4056 Iowa City, IA 52243 (319) 337-1357

MCAT scores may be released directly to the American Medical College Application Service (AMCAS) at the time of the test. If released, AMCAS will automatically forward the two most recent MCAT scores with application materials to AMCAS-participating schools to which the applicant applies. Please note, however, that AMCAS will not forward scores from pre-1991 MCAT administrations. At the time of the test, examinees may also designate six non-AMCAS institutions (i.e., non-AMCAS allopathic medical schools, schools of osteopathic, podiatric and veterinary medicine) as score recipients at no cost.

MCAT QUESTIONS & ANSWERS

• Which is more important, a good GPA from a respected school, or a good MCAT score?

The MCAT is inching ahead of GPA/School, with the Verbal Reasoning section inching ahead of the Physical Sciences and the Biological Sciences.

• How would you rate the relative importance of each subtest on the MCAT, as viewed by the average admissions committee?

On a scale of 1-15, with 15 being the most important subtest, I'd give Verbal Reasoning a 15, Physical and Biological Sciences a 14, and the Writing Sample a 2.

• Do admission committees add up my individual subtest scores to get a total MCAT score?

No, I have never heard of such a thing being done.

• I've released two sets of recent MCAT scores. How do admissions committees use this information? Do they take the average? Do they look at the high score? Do they look at the more recent score?

They look at both scores. There is no generic formula used to evaluate multiple MCAT scores.

• **I did poorly on the MCAT the first time, but did much better the second time. Should I release both scores?**

The majority opinion on this one is "yes", but most folks in the know admit that they are not sure. Of course, the specifics of your individual application should also be considered.

• **What are the important differences between the MCAT and the tests I've taken in the sciences?**

The MCAT is more conceptual and far less numeric (On average, less than five questions on the entire MCAT require more than a couple of multiplications, divisions, additions, or subtractions). The test stresses relationships, proportions, consequences, and fundamental principles. Most MCAT questions in the Sciences present novel information to you in the form of passages. You will be expected to integrate this new information with material you already have mastered in order to arrive at the correct answer.

• **What is the best way to prepare?**

Whether you take a prep course or not there are four essentials.

One - Learn all you can about the MCAT.
Two - Get complete and appropriate reference materials.
Three - Use a source of high quality practice tests.
Four - Put in the time.

Scoring of the Writing Sample

Each of your essays will be read and scored by two different readers on a six-point scale. The readers are looking for your ability to organize an answer, explain the statement, develop a central concept, synthesize conflicting concepts and ideas, and express yourself clearly and correctly.

Essays receiving scores that differ by more than one point will be evaluated by a third reader who determines the total score for the paper. Scoring is done holistically; the essay is considered as a unit without separable aspects. A single score is assigned to an essay based on the quality of the writing as a whole.

Each essay is judged on its overall effectiveness after the readers determine whether all three writing tasks have been addressed. Mistakes are expected on essays because candidates are writing under timed conditions. Minor grammatical errors will not overly affect the paper's evaluation. The thoroughness, depth, and clarity of ideas presented in the essay will determine the score.

The essay topics will not be controversial subjects such as religion or politics, nor will they be medical topics or topics requiring prior knowledge. The essays are scored on a scale of 1 to 6 (see table on next page). This numerical score is then converted to a letter score.

Failure to respond to any one of the three writing tasks will reduce your score by three points. Copies of your essays will be sent to those medical schools that request them.

Criteria for Scoring Writing Samples

Numerical Score	Letter Score	All 3 Tasks Addressed	Quality of Essay
1	J - K	No - may entirely fail to address the topic	Marked problems with organization and mechanics that make the language very difficult to follow.
2	L - M	No - seriously neglects or distorts one or more of the writing tasks	Problems with organization and analysis of the topic. They may contain recurrent mechanical errors resulting in language that is occasionally difficult to follow.
3	N - O	No - neglects or distorts one or more of the writing tasks or presents only a minimal treatment of the topic	Some clarity of thought shown, but may be simplistic. Problems in organization may be evident. The essays demonstrate a basic control of vocabulary and sentence structure, but the language may not effectively communicate the writer's ideas.
4	P - Q	Yes - moderate treatment of each	Shows clarity of thought, but they may lack complexity. Demonstration of coherent organization although some digressions may be evident. The writing shows an overall control of vocabulary and sentence structure.
5	R - S	Yes - substantial treatment of each	Shows some depth of thought, coherent organization, and control of vocabulary and sentence structure.
6	T	Yes - thorough treatment of each	Shows depth and complexity of thought, focused and coherent organization, and a superior control of vocabulary and sentence structure.

NOTES

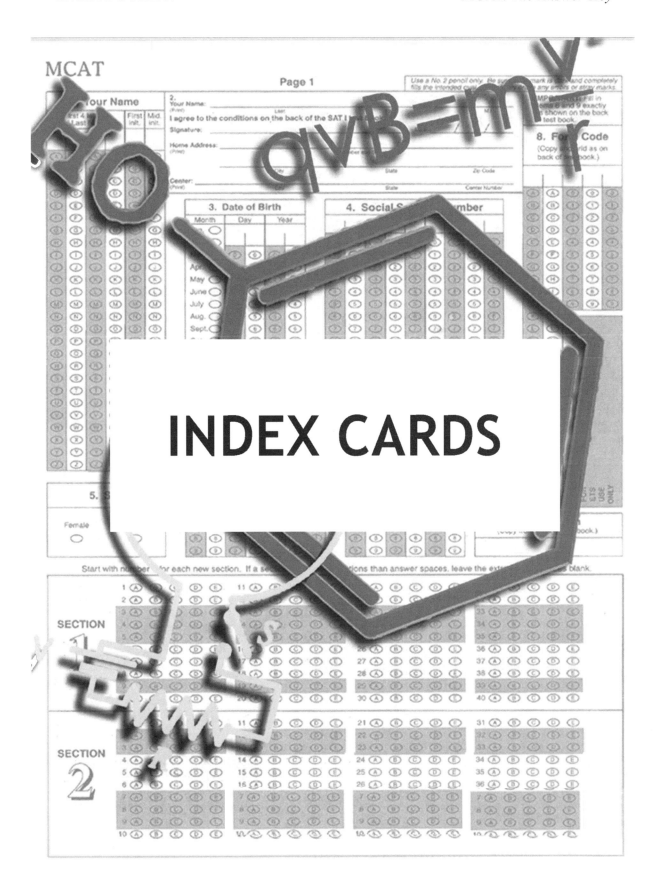

THE CELLS: Enzyme Regulation

ALLOSTERIC EFFECT: is experienced by an enzyme that has multiple reaction sites on it. When a ligand is bound to one of these reactive sites, it forces a conformational change in the structure of the enzyme that renders all the other reaction sites from binding other ligands/substrates.

FEEDBACK INHIBITIONS: end product inhibits any further activity of the enzyme. Feedback inhibition is sensitive to the concentration of the end product of a reaction.

COMPETITIVE INHIBITIONS: substrate and inhibitor both bind to the same active site. This process may be reversed by increasing the concentration of the substrare.

NON-COMPETITIVE INHIBITIONS: substrate and inhibitor have different binding sites on the same enzyme. Non-competitive inhibition cannot be reversed by increasing the concentration of the substrate.

THE CELLS: Organelles

ORGANELLE	FUNCTION(s)
Nucleus	The home of the DNA.
Nucleolus	Region within the nucleus where rRNA is synthesized
Ribsosomes	Decodes mRNA and synthesizes proteins.
Endoplasmic Reticulum	Used for intracellular transportation.
Rough	ER Complex of ER and ribosomes
Smooth	ER Participates in the synthesis of lipids.
Mitochondria	Sythesizes ATP molecules via cell respiration
Golgi body	Packages newly synthesized proteins by adding sugar or lipid molecules to them; produces vesicles.
Lysosomes	Participates in intracellular digestion by releasing lytic enzymes.
Centrioles	Participates in cell division by producing spindle fibers

THE CELLS: Enzymes

Enzymes are biological catalysts that modify the rate of reactions in cells. Enzymes are specific to the substrates that they interact with ("lock and key" model).

STRUCTURE: All enzymes are complex proteins with one or more active sites. Substrate react with enzyme to form enzyme-substrate complex at active site. Sometimes enzymes are formed in association with non-protein molecules such as vitamins. Non-protein molecules are also referred to as coenzymes.

Factors That Affect Enzymes' Biological Activities:

1. **Temperature:** As temperature increases, the enzyme catalyzed reaction rate also increase. However, at relatively high temperature enzymes denature. Most enzymes denature at temperature around 40°C.
2. **pH:** All enzymes operate at its optimum pH. Most enzymes prefer an ambient pH that is similar to the physiological pH (apprx. 7.4). The function of the enzyme varies according to the pH. Acidic pH tend to denature most enzymes.

THE CELLS: Biochemistry

PROTEINS

PROTEINS: contain carbon, hydrogen, nitrogen, and oxygen. The building blocks of all proteins are 20 known amino acids. An amino acid contains an amino group (NH_2) and a carboxyl group (COOH). Proteins are polypeptide chains made of amino acids bonded to each other via the peptide bond.

Peptide bonds are formed as result of dehydration synthesis.

Proteins serve in numerous capacities in humans. Proteins act as hormones and enzymes. They also serve as structural molecules in cell membranes.

THE CELLS: Biochemistry

VITAMINS

Vitamins are organic compounds. Vitamins often act as coenzymes in humans.

FAT SOLUABLE VITAMINS:
- **Vitamin A**: deficiency causes poor vision.
- **Vitamin D**: enhances absorption of calcium by bones. Deficiency causes Rickets.
- **Vitamin E**: often perceived to be important for normal reproduction.
- **Vitamin K**: is required for normal blood clotting.

WATER SOLUAQBLE VITAMINS:
- **Thiamine (B_1)**: deficiency results in beriberi. Required for normal functioning of the nervous system.
- **Riboflavin (B_2)**: required for certain chemical reactions in humans.
- **Niacin**: deficiency leads to pellagra. Niacin acts as the functional group in NAD and NADP.
- **Vitamin C:** required for normal collogen synthesis. Deficiency causes Scurvy.

GENETICS: Nucleotides

DNA: is composed of long, repeating chain of nucleotides.

Nucleotides are composed of:
- A phosphate group
- 5 carbon sugar – deoxyribose
- A nitrogenous base

The four nitrogenous bases are: adenine, thymine, guanine, and cytosine.

GENETICS: CONCEPTS

- **Dominance**: is the principle that defines the expression of one allele over another for a given trait (ex: black hair is dominant over brown hair).
- **Incomplete Dominance**: is the principle that defines the partial expression of a dominant allele over a recessive allele (ex: In certain flowers, the color pink results from partial expression of the color red).
- **Codominance**: is the principle that defines expression of both alleles in an individual (ex: the alleles red and white are both expressed in cows to produce a coat color called roan).
- **Segregation**: is the processes in which alleles are separated from each other when gametes are formed (diploid 2N to haploid N).
- **Independent Assortment**: is the principle that states that the segregation of the alleles of one trait is independent of the segregation of any of the others.
- **Gene Linkage**: states that alleles of different traits located on the same chromosome maybe inherited together.

MEIOSIS: Ovum

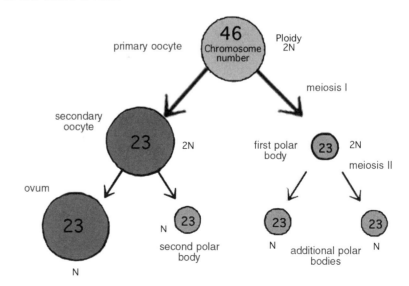

MEIOSIS: Sperm Cells

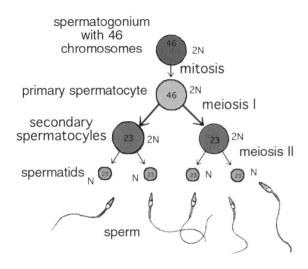

spermatogonium with 46 chromosomes

46 2N

mitosis

primary spermatocyte 46 2N

meiosis I

secondary spermatocyles 23 2N   23 2N

meiosis II

spermatids 23 N   N 23   23 N   N 23 N

sperm

MICROBIOLOGY: Viral Infection Cycles

LYTIC INFECTION

- Virus binds to receptors on host cell membranes
- Injects viral nucleic acid
- Viral replication takes place in host cells (replication takes place only once)
- New virus particles are released when host cells lysis

LYSOGENIC INFECTION

- Virus binds to receptors on host cell membranes
- Injects viral nucleic acid
- Viral DNA integrates into host chromosomes
- Replication of both viral and host DNA take place
- Viral genome is replicated many times before host cells lyse

MICROBIOLOGY: Bacteria

CLASSIFICATION OF BACTERIA

- **OBLIGATE AEROBES**: cannot survive without oxygen.

- **OBLIGATE ANAEROBES**: cannot survive in an environment rich in oxygen.

- **FACULTATIVE ANAEROBES**: can survive in an environment that may be rich or void of oxygen.

Obligate and facultative anaerobes produce alcohol via fermentation under anaerobic condition.

MICROBIOLOGY: Bacteria

SUMMARY: SHAPES OF BACTERIA

SHAPE	NAME
Rod-shaped	Bacillus (singular); bacilli (plural)
Round	Coccus (singular); cocci(plural)
Spiral-shaped	Spirillum (singular); spirilla (plural)

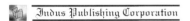
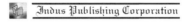

BIOLOGY: Sex Linked Traits

Sex-linked traits and other hereditary aberrations

Genotype: Female: XX   Male: XY

X chromosome is larger in size than the Y chromosome. As a result,
     it carries additional genetic traits other than genes that determine
     the sex of an individual.

Sex-linked traits (males are mostly affected) (X-Linked Disorders)

- Color blindness
- Hemophilia
- Baldness

Down's Syndrome: extra chromosome #21

Turner's Syndrome: XO (affects females only)

Klinefelter Syndrome: XXY (affects males only)

AUTONOMOUS NERVOUS SYSTEM

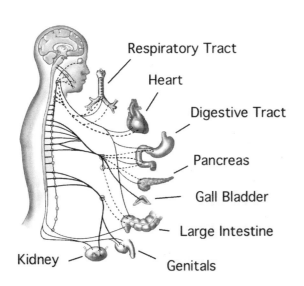

Respiratory Tract

Heart

Digestive Tract

Pancreas

Gall Bladder

Large Intestine

Kidney   Genitals

GENETICS: Nature Of Gene Control

REPRESSOR PROTEINS: prevent RNA polymerases from binding to DNA
     (negative control). Example: Lactose Metabolism in *E. Coli*

ACTIVATOR PROTEINS: promotes greater binding of RNA polymerases
     to DNA (positive control). Example: Nitrogen metabolism in
     prokaryotes

The enhanced or reduced binding of RNA polymerases to DNA are often
     mediated by control agents such as hormones.

Control agents may bind to **promoter sequence** located at the start
     of a gene or to the **operator sequence** located between the
     promoter and the start of a gene.

OPERON: is the sequence of bases that consists of the promoter,
     the operator, and the gene(s) that code a specific protein.

BLOOD WATER CONTENT

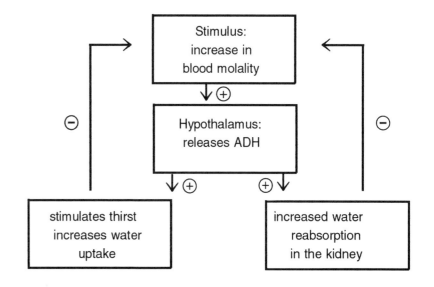

Stimulus:
increase in
blood molality

$\ominus$

$\downarrow \oplus$

Hypothalamus:
releases ADH

$\ominus$

$\downarrow \oplus$ $\oplus \downarrow$

stimulates thirst
increases water
uptake

increased water
reabsorption
in the kidney

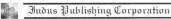

Blood Flow Through The Heart

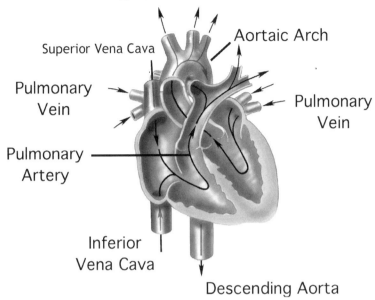

Superior Vena Cava

Aortaic Arch

Pulmonary Vein

Pulmonary Vein

Pulmonary Artery

Inferior Vena Cava

Descending Aorta

THE NERVOUS SYSTEM

THE COMPONENTS OF THE NERVOUS SYSTEM

NEURONS: or nerve cells are basis of the nervous systems.
   All nerve cells are composed of three basic structures:
      axon, dendrites, and the soma (cell body).

There are three types of neurons:
   • **SENSORY NEURONS:** are responsible for transmitting impulses from
      receptors to the Central Nervous System (CNS).
   • **MOTOR NEURONS:** are responsible for transmitting messages from the
      CNS to the effectors such as the muscles and glands.
   • **INTERNEURONS:** are only found in the CNS and their primary function
      is to act as liaisons between sensory and motor neurons.

DIRECTION OF IMPULSE CONDUCTION: Sensory Neurons → Interneuron
      → Motor Neurons

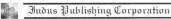

CENTRAL NERVOUS SYSTEM

THE BRAIN: Functions
   • **CEREBRUM**: consists of right and left hemispheres, five lobes (frontal,
      temporal, parietal, occipital, and insula) and an outer cortex (made
      of gray matter). Plays a significant role in memory and reasoning
      processes, learning "conditioned behaviors."
   • **DIENCEPHALON**: consists of the thalamus (directs sensory impulses
      to the cerebral cortex) and the hypothalamus (maintains general
      homeostasis, controls pituitary gland).
   • **BRAIN STEM**: consists of the following: midbrain (controls eye and ear
      reflexes, pons (connects various parts of the brain), and the medulla
      oblongata (regulates the respiratory center, heart rate, and vascular activities).
   • **CEREBELLUM**: coordinates motor activities (skeletal muscle
      movements and balance).
   • **SPINAL CORD**: consists of three meningeal: dura mater
      (outermost), arachnoid (middle), and the pia mater (innermost).

THE NERVOUS SYSTEM: PERIPHERAL NERVOUS SYSTEM
   PNS consist of all the nerves that innervate various parts of the body
   that lie entirely outside the central nervous system.

   • **SOMATIC NERVOUS SYSTEM:** is composed of neurons that innervate
      voluntary muscles.
   • **AUTONOMIC NERVOUS SYSTEM:** consists of neurons that innervate organs
      composed of smooth or cardiac muscles (eg: heart, the digestive tract).
   • **PARASYMPATHETIC NERVOUS SYSTEM:** usually induce inhibitory
      responses in the body.
      (MAJOR EXCEPTION: Parasympathetic nerves stimulate muscles in the
         digestive tract and erection of the penis.
      • The primary neurotransmitter associated with parasympathetic nerves
         is acetylcholine.
   • **SYMPATHETIC NERVOUS SYSTEM:** usually induce excitatory responses
      in the body.
      • The primary neurotransmitters associated with sympathetic nerves
         are norepinephrine and acetylcholine.

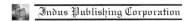

SYMPATHETIC VS PARASYMPATHETIC

SYMPATHETIC NERVOUS SYSTEM (fight or flight):
- Increases heart rate, blood circulation to vital organs, dilates pupil
- Promotes vasoconstriction in skin, promotes piloerection
- Generates an increase in metabolic rate
- Decreases activity of the digestive tract

PARASYMPATHETIC NERVOUS SYSTEM
- Simulates vagus nerve, decreases heart rate, increases activity of the digestive tract

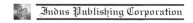

THE NERVOUS SYSTEM

THE BRAIN: Functions

CEREBELLUM:
Coordinates motor activities (skeletal muscle movements). Helps maintain proper balance and posture.

CEREBRUM:
Sensory impulses are processed here. Cerebrum plays an important role in memory and reasoning processes. Also plays a significant role in learning "conditioned behaviors."

MEDULLA:
Controls involuntary activities including breathing, blood pressure, movements of the digestive organs, sneezing, and heartbeat.

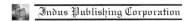

CENTRAL NERVOUS SYSTEM: The Brain

- **THALAMUS**: directs sensory impulses to the cerebral cortex.

- **HYPOTHALAMUS**: maintains general homeostasis; controls the pituitary gland.

- **MIDBRAIN**: controls eye and ear reflexes.

- **PONS**: connects various parts of the brain.

- **MEDULLA OBLONGATA**: is attached to the spinal cord; regulates the respiratory center, heart rate, and vasomotor activities.

- **CEREBELLUM**: is responsible for coordination, muscle tone, and balance.

- **SPINAL CORD**: conducts sensory and motor impulses to and from brain; mediates reflex activities.

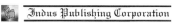

THE NERVOUS SYSTEM

The REFLEX ARC

The reflex arc consists of the following:

sensory receptor on dendrite (dorsal root ganglion) → dorsal root ganglion cell body → axon of the dorsal root ganglion → dorsal horn of spinal cord → dendrite of ventral horn motor cell (sometimes an interneuron may be involved) → ventral motor cell body → axon of the ventral root ganglion → effector organ/tissue

CIRCULATORY SYSTEM: Blood

Blood is the basis of the circulatory system in the human. Blood is defined as a soft tissue composed of fluid and formed elements. Blood plays an important role in maintaining homeostasis throughout the human body.

PLASMA: is composed of water and dissolved ions such as sodium and potassium. In addition, hormones, nutrients, antibodies, enzymes, clotting factors, and waste products are also found dissolved in the plasma.

RED BLOOD CELLS (Erythrocytes): are hemoglobin containing cells that transport oxygen to all cells in the body. Mature RBCs are disk-shaped and lack nucleus.

WHITE BLOOD CELLS (Leukocytes): are a collection of variety of cells that work together to form the immune system of the human body.
- **Five types of WBC**: Neutrophil, Eosinophil, Basophil, Lymphocyte, and Monocyte.

PLATELETS: are cell fragments that play a critical role in the blood clotting process.

CIRCULATORY SYSTEM: Blood Types

BLOOD TYPES

Blood Type	Genotype	Legend
A	$I^A I^A$ / $I^A i$	I^A = allele for protein A
B	$I^B I^B$ / $I^B i$	I^B = allele for protein B
AB	$I^A I^B$	i = no allele is present (A or B)
O	ii	

The genotype $I^A I^B$ is an example of codominance.

CIRCULATORY SYSTEM

Circulatory System Related Formulas

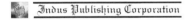

BLOOD FLOW (F) = $\dfrac{\text{difference in blood pressure between two points (DP)}}{\text{Peripheral resistance (R)}}$

MEAN ARTERIAL PRESSURE = diastolic pressure + (pulse pressure/3)
pulse pressure = the difference between the systolic and diastolic pressures.

CARDIAC OUTPUT = Stroke volume (ml/beat) X heart rate (beats per min)

BLOOD PRESSURE = Cardiac output X Peripheral resistance

DEVELOPMENTAL BIOLOGY

ENDODERM
GI Tract, inner lining of respiratory tract, esophagus, stomach small intestine, large intestine, pancreas, gall bladder, liver, thyroid gland, trachea, bronchi, bronchioles, and alveoli

ECTODERM
epidermis, eye, CNS

MESODERM
excretory system, reproductive system, musculoskeletal system, circulatory system, and PNS

THE DIGESTIVE SYSTEM

THE DIGESTIVE SYSTEM: the Small Intestine and the Large Intestine

THE SMALL IINTESTINE: is a long tube that is located in the lower region of the G.I. tract. Partially digested food from the stomach is completely digested in the small intestine. The small intestine works in tandem with accessory digestive structures including the pancreas and the gall bladder to breakdown major macromolecules. The pancreas releases a proteolvtic enzyme called trypsin. Bile is synthesized in the liver and released from the gall bladder.

ABSORPTION IN THE SMALL IINTESTINE: the small intestine wall contains finger-like projections called villi. Villi increase the surface area in the small intestine which improve the rate of absorption. Fatty acids and glycerol are absorbed through structures known as lacteals.

THE LARGE INTESTINE: is the site where H_2O and excess alkaline fluid released in the small intestine are reabsorbed back into the body. Critical vitamins and essential amino acids are also synthesized by mutualistic bacterial colonies that reside in the large intestine.

THE DIGESTIVE SYSTEM

SUMMARY - Chemical Digestion

Organs/Glands	Enzymes	Macromolecule Digested
Mouth	Amylase	Starch
Stomach	Pepsin	Protein
Small Intestine		
Intestinal glands	Lactase	Lactose
	Maltase	Maltose
	Sucrase	Sucrose
Pancreas	Trypsin	Protein
Gall Bladder	Bile	Lipids (emulsified)

END PRODUCTS: Protein → amino acids
Disaccharides/Polysaccharides→monosaccharides
Lipids→1 glycerol + 3 fatty acids

THE DIGESTIVE SYSTEM

THE DIGESTIVE SYSTEM: Mouth, Esophagus, and the Stomach

MOUTH: Ingestion of food occurs in the oral cavity. Mechanical breakdown (chewing) of food takes place here. The chemical digestion of carbohydrate is initiated when salivary glands release the enzyme amylase.

ESOPHAGUS: After food is swallowed, it moves into the esophagus. The process of peristalsis propels the swallowed food through the upper G.I. tract into the stomach.

STOMACH: is a muscular organ where chemical digestion of protein is initiated. The swallowed food is liquefied to gelatinous mass called chyme. The gastric glands release a host of proteolytic enzymes and hydrochloric acid (HCl). The release of HCl results in the pH of the stomach to be extremely acidic (pH=2).

ENDOCRINE SYSTEM: Endocrine Glands

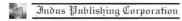
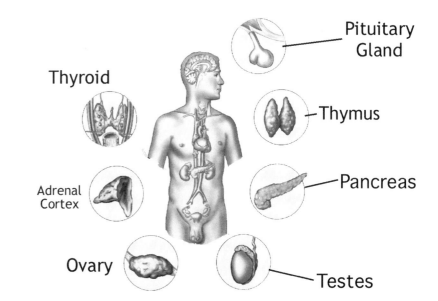

THE ENDOCRINE SYSTEM

GLAND	HORMONES(S)	EFFECTS
Adrenal cortex	Glucocorticoids	Promotes metabolic activities
	Mineralocorticoids	Regulates electrolytes and water content
Pancreas	Insulin	Regulates cellular intake of glucose
	Glucagon	Stimulates liver to release stored glucose
Thymus	Thymosin	Affects T-lymphocyte development
Ovary	Estrogen	Stimulates growth of primary sex organs and secondary sex characteristics in females
	Progesterone	Prepares uterine lining for possible pregnancy
Testes	Testosterone	Stimulates growth of primary sex organs and secondary sex characteristics in males

- Hormones may be proteins or steroids.
- A process called a negative feedback system regulates the release of most hormones.

THE MUSCULAR SYSTEM

THE SLIDING FILAMENT MODEL OF CONTRACTION

1. Nervous stimulus takes place.
2. Acetylcholine is released at neuromuscular junction.
3. Ca^{+2} ions are released from the sarcoplasmic reticulum.
4. Ca^{+2} ions bind to troponin molecules causing them to physically shift on the actin myofilaments.
5. Actin is ready to bind myosin heads when troponin molecules shift.
6. ATP molecules are hydrolyzed to ADP and Pi and myosin heads attach to actin.
7. As a result of cross bridge attachments between myosin and actin, the myosin heads pull on the actin (the power stroke) thus allowing the two myofilaments to slide past each other.
8. Cross bridge detachment occurs when new ATP molecules attach to myosin heads.
9. Cross bridge detachment returns the myosin to its original position, thus ending muscle contraction.

THE MUSCULAR SYSTEM

THE STRUCTURE OF STRIATED MUSCLE CELLS

A muscle fiber is composed of a single muscle cell that is surrounded by a membrane called the sarcolemma. Usually several nuclei are present in a single muscle cell. Each muscle fiber is composed of numerous myofilaments called myosin and actin.

The myofilaments display dark and light areas/bands – "I" and "A" bands respectively. The "I" band is bisected by the "Z" line while the "A" band is bisected by the "M" line. "A" band is also interrupted in the midsection by another light strip termed the "H" zone.

A sarcomere is a segment of the muscle fiber between two successive Z lines.

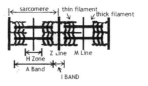

THE MUSCULAR SYSTEM

MUSCLE TYPE	CHARACTERISTICS	LOCATION
Skeletal	Striated & Voluntary	Skeletal muscles (eg: biceps)
Smooth	Non-striated & Involuntary	Muscles controlled by the autonomic nervous system (eg: walls of the digestive tract and blood vessels).
Cardiac	Striated & Involuntary	Heart

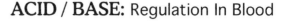
PHYSIOLOGY OF THE HEART

BRADYCARDIA: lower than normal heart rate (60 beats per minute or less)

TACHYCARDIA: higher than normal heart rate (100 beats per minute or more)

EXTRASYSTOLE: premature heart beat

NORMAL HEART SOUNDS:
    LUBB: indicates closing of artrioventricular vaves
    DUPP: indicates closing of semilunar valves.
    STROKE VOLUME: amount of blood pumped with each beat.

ACID / BASE: Regulation In Blood

$$CO_2 + H_2O \rightleftharpoons H_2CO_3 \rightleftharpoons HCO_3^- + H^+$$
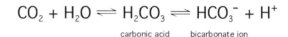
             carbonic acid   bicarbonate ion

During hyperventilation, the reaction shifts to the left.

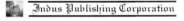
THE RESPIRATORY SYSTEM

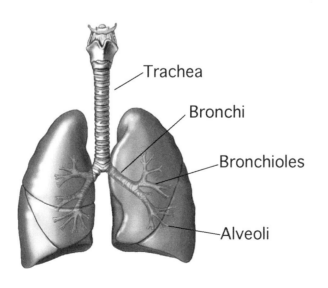

Trachea

Bronchi

Bronchioles

Alveoli

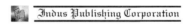
THE RESPIRATORY SYSTEM

THE RESPIRATORY SYSTEM: is composed of the following structures:
- **NASAL CAVITY:** is located within the nose and exposed to the outside via the nostrils. Nasal cavity is the first stop of inspired air in humans.
- **PHARYNX:** is an area where the nasal cavity and the oral cavity combine to form a distinct air passage. A flap of tissue called the epiglottis separates the pharynx from the trachea.
- **TRACHEA:** is a tube that connects the pharynx with the bronchi. The trachea is prevented from collapsing by cartilage rings that surround the tube.
- **BRONCHI:** are part of the respiratory tract that enter the lungs. The end of trachea divides into two bronchi, one entering the left lung and one entering the right lung. Like the trachea, each stem of the bronchi also contains cartilage rings.
- **BRONCHIOLES:** are small subdivisions of the bronchi. Bronchiolar walls are lined with mucous membrane, but they lack cartilage rings.
- **ALVEOLI:** are clusters of air sacs at the end of bronchioles where gases are exchanged.

THE SKELETAL SYSTEM: Bones

Human bones are composed of collagen and hydroxyappetite (a complex made of Ca^{+2} and inorganic phosphate).

Spongy bones contain either red or yellow marrow.

Compact bones have an internal canal system called the Haversian canals, which are used to transport nutrients to various parts of the bone.

OSTEOBLAST: are cells that assist in building up bones by concentration Ca^{+2} complex.

OSTEOCLAST: are cells that assist in breaking down bones.

OSTEOCYTES: are mature bone cells.

THE SPINAL NERVE

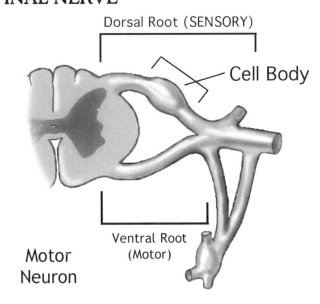

Dorsal Root (SENSORY)

Cell Body

Ventral Root (Motor)

Motor Neuron

THE RESPIRATORY SYSTEM

THE PROCESS OF BREATHING

The process of breathing is highly dependent on the actions of the diaphragm and the rib cage. The movement of the muscle called the diaphragm and rib cage accounts for the passive movement of air in and out of the lungs.

INHALATION: is the process of breathing in of air. During inhalation, the dome shaped diaphragm contracts increasing the thoracic volume. As a result, a negative pressure relative to the atmospheric pressure is created in the lungs. In response to the negative pressure, air rushes into the lungs. Exhalation is the expulsion of air from the lungs. During exhalation, diaphragm relaxes to effectively reduce the thoracic volume. Consequently, the pressure inside the lungs rises. As a result, air rushes out of the lungs and into the external environment.

REGULATION: Respiration is regulated from the respiratory center in the medulla. Phrenic nerve is responsible for regulating the rate of contraction of diaphragm.

THE BRAIN

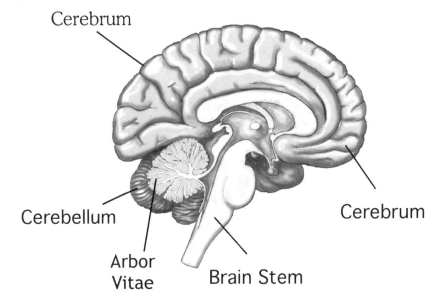

Cerebrum

Cerebellum

Cerebrum

Arbor Vitae

Brain Stem

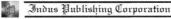

THE NEPHRON

Glomerulus

Proximal Convulated Tubules

Distal Convulated Tubules

Collecting Duct

Loop Of Henle

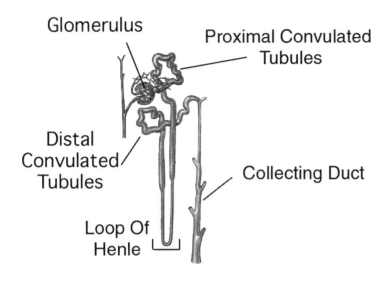

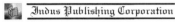

THE URINARY SYSTEM: Renal Physiology

BLOOD SUPPLY TO THE NEPHRON:

• **RENAL ARTERY** supplies oxygenated blood to the kidney.

• **AFFERENT ARTERIOLE** enters Bowman's capsule.

• **GLOMERULUS** is a coil of capillaries where filtration takes place.

• **PERITUBULAR CAPILLARIES** surround the nephron and is the site of major reabsorption.

• **FILTRATION**: takes place at the glomerulus.

• **REABSORPTION**: takes place in the Proximal Convoluted Tubule, the loop of Henle, the Distal Convoluted Tubule, and the Collecting Duct (water only).

• **SECRETION**: takes place in the PCT, the loop of Henle, and the DCT.

ANATOMY: Blood Vessels

Most blood vessels are composed of three layers of tissues:

ENDOTHELIUM (innermost): a middle layer of elastic connective tissue and an outer layer.
ASCENDING AORTA: gives rise to the left and right coronary arteries.
AORTIC ARCH: gives rise to the brachiocephalic trunk, left common carotid artery and the left subclavian artery.

VASOCONSTRICTION: decrease in diameter of the blood vessel (the velocity of the blood flow increases).

VASODILATION: increase in the diameter of the blood vessel (the velocity of the blood flow decreases).

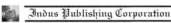

THE URINARY SYSTEM: Renal Physiology

REGULATORY ACTIVITIES IN THE KIDNEY:
The concentration of electrolytes such as sodium, calcium, potassium, chloride, and phosphate in the body are regulated by the kidney.

IMPORTANT RENAL REGULATORY HORMONES:
• **ALDOSTERONE**: promotes reabsorption of Na^+ and secretion of K^+ in the distal convoluted tubule (DCT).
• **CALCITONIN**: decreases the concentration of Ca^{+2} in the blood.
• **PARATHYROID HORMONE**: increases the concentration of Ca^{+2} in the blood.

ACIDS & BASES: Characteristics

ACIDS
- Strong acids react with strong bases to form water and a salt (neutralization reaction).
- Acids react with certain metals to produce hydrogen gas.
- Acids cause color changes in solution in the presence of an indicator.
- Aqueous acidic solutions conduct electricity.
- Acids are sour in test.
- Strong acids ionize more than weak acids in solution.

BASES
- Strong bases react with strong acids to form water and a salt (neutralization reaction).
- Aqueous basic solutions conduct electricity.
- Bases cause color changes in solution in the presence of an indicator.
- Bases are slippery in feeling.
- Strong bases ionize more than weak bases in solution.

ACIDS & BASES: Amphoteric Substances

AMPHOTEC SUBSTANCES: are chemical substances that can acts as an acid or a base. In other words, amphoteric substances can both donate or accept a proton.

$$H_2O + NH_3 \longleftrightarrow NH_4^+ + OH^-$$
acid base   acid   base

$$H_2O + HNO_3 \longleftrightarrow H_3O^+ + NO3^-$$
base acid   acid   base

Example of H_2O acting as both an acid and a base in two separate reactions.

Clue: Amphoteric substances can be easily spotted. All amphoteric substances have at least one hydrogen (H) and a negative charge as part of its overall structure.

ACIDS & BASES: Definitions Of Acids & Bases

BRONSTED-LOWRY ACIDS: are defined as chemical compounds which donate proton(s).
$$NH_3 + H_2O \longrightarrow NH_4^+ + OH^-$$
(H_2O is the Bronsted acid since it donates a proton to NH_3)

BRONSTED-LOWRY BASES: are defined as chemical compounds which accept proton(s).
$$NH_3 + H_2O \longrightarrow NH_4^+ + OH^-$$ an electron pair.

LEWIS BASES: are defined as chemical compounds which donate an electron pair.

AMPHOTERIC SUBSTANCES: can act as both an acid or a base depending on the chemical reaction.

In this reaction water acts as an acid: H_2O (acid) $+ NH_3 \longrightarrow NH_4^+ + OH^-$

In this reaction water acts as a base: H_2O (base) $+ HNO_3 \longrightarrow H_3O^+ + NO_3^-$

(NH_3 is the Bronsted base since it accepts a proton from H_2O)

Lewis Acids: are defined as chemical compounds which accept electrons.

ACIDS & BASES: Conjugate Acid-Base Pairs

CONJUGATE ACID-BASE PAIRS: are based on the principal that all acid-base reactions are reversible.

CONJUGATE ACID-BASE PAIRS: are two chemical substances (ex: ions) whose structure differ by only one H+ ion.

$$HCl + H_2O \longrightarrow H_3O+ + Cl^-$$

$$Acid_1 + Base_2 \longrightarrow Acid_2 + Base_1$$

Conjugate acid-base pairs: HCl and Cl^-
Conjugate acid-base pairs: H_2O and H_3O^+

ACIDS & BASES: Acid-Base Titration

ACID-BASE TITRATION: is the process of gradually adding measured volumes of an acid or base of known concentration (molarity) to an acid or base of unknown concentration (molarity) until neutralization occurs.

END POINT or EQUIVALENCE POINT: is the point at which stoichiometrically equivalent quantities of acid and base have reacted with each other during a titration.

Unknown molarity of an acid or base can be calculated by using the following formula:

Volume Acid X Molarity Acid = Volume Base X Molarity Base

Moles of Acid = Volume of Acid (L) X Molarity of Acid

Moles of Base = Volume of Base (L) X Molarity of Base

ACIDS & BASES: Ionization Constant

IONIZATION CONSTANT OF BASES (K_b)

IONIZATION CONSTANT: represents a base's ability to ionize in solution. The greater the K_b of a base, the larger the amount of ionization. Therefore, a base with a $K_b = 1 \times 10^6$ is stronger than a base with a $K_b = 1 \times 10^3$. In the same manner, a base with a $K_b = 1 \times 10^3$ is stronger than a base with a $K_b = 1 \times 10^{-3}$.

$$BOH \rightarrow B^+ + OH^- \text{ where BOH = undissociated base}$$
$$B^+ = \text{metal ion}$$
$$OH^- = \text{base}$$

$$\text{Ionization Constant} = K_b = \frac{[B^+][OH^-]}{[BOH]}$$

Temperature may affect the K_b value of a base.

ACTIVATION ENERGY
(exothermic reaction)

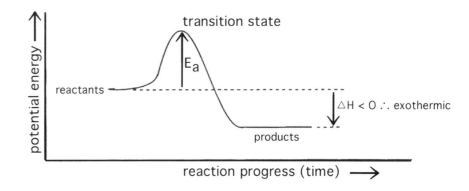

E_a = activation energy
ΔH = change in potential energy

ACIDITY TREND
(the periodic table)

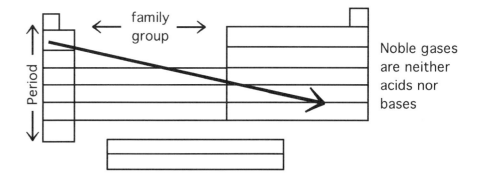

Noble gases are neither acids nor bases

ACIDS & BASES: Titration Curve

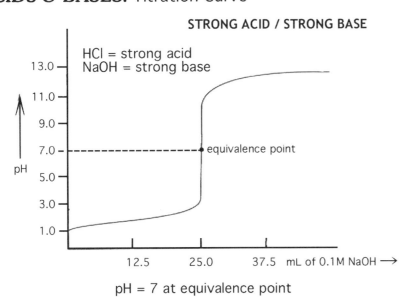

STRONG ACID / STRONG BASE

HCl = strong acid
NaOH = strong base

pH = 7 at equivalence point

ACIDS & BASES: Titration Curve

STRONG ACID / WEAK BASE

HCl = strong acid
CH_3COO^- = weak base

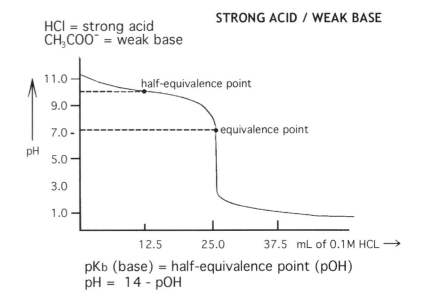

pK_b (base) = half-equivalence point (pOH)
pH = 14 - pOH

ACIDS & BASES: Titration Curve - Diprotic Acid

WEAK ACID / STRONG BASE

H_2SO_4 = weak acid
NaOH = strong base

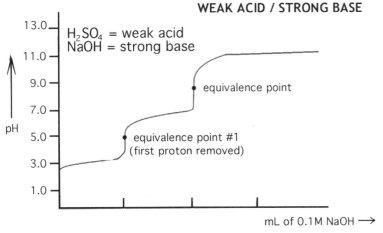

Titration #1: $H_2SO_4 \longrightarrow H^+ + HSO_4^-$
Titration #2: $HSO_4^- \longrightarrow H^+ + SO_4^{-2}$

ACIDS & BASES: Titration Curve

WEAK ACID / STRONG BASE

HF = weak acid
NaOH = strong base

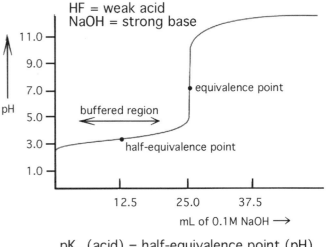

pK_a (acid) = half-equivalence point (pH)

ATOMIC STRUCTURE: Subshells

THE ORDER IN WHICH THEY ARE FILLED

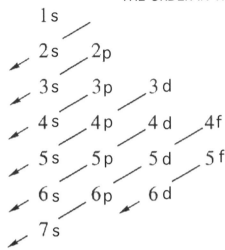

ATOMIC STRUCTURE: Mass Number

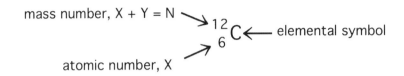

X = number of protons (atomic number)
Y = number of neutrons
N = number of protons + number of neutrons (mass number)

Isotopes of the same element defer in their mass numbers.
(The number of neutrons vary, but the number of protons remain the same)

ACIDS & BASES: pH Scale

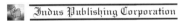

acidic   basic

←———————— neutral ————————→

0.0 1.0 2.0 3.0 4.0 5.0 6.0 7.0 8.0 9.0 10.0 11.0 12.0 13.0 14.0

$$pH = [H^+]$$

$$pOH = [OH^-]$$

ATOMIC STRUCTURE: Radioactive Decay

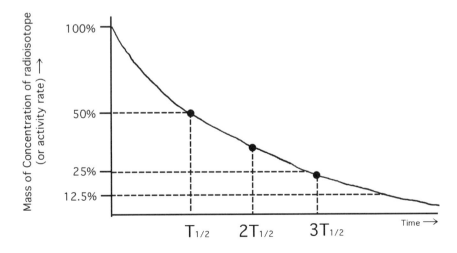

ATOMIC STRUCTURE: Geometric Family

SQUARE PRYAMID

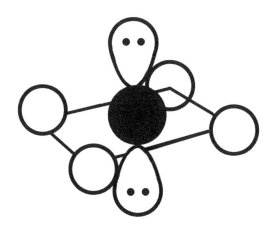

ATOMIC STRUCTURE: Geometric Family

Octahedral

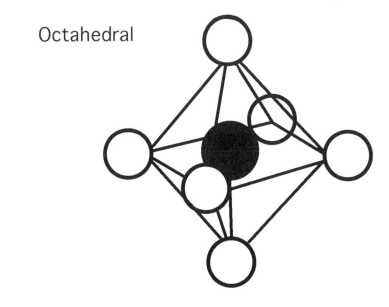

ATOMIC STRUCTURE: Geometric Family

TRIGONAL BIPYRAMID

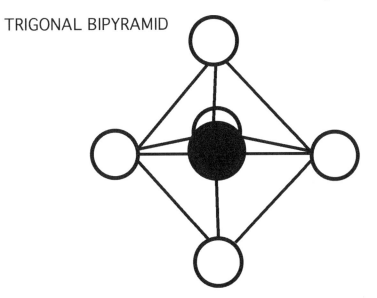

ATOMIC STRUCTURE: Geometric Family

LINEAR

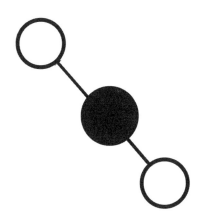

ATOMIC STRUCTURE: Geometric Family

SEE-SAW

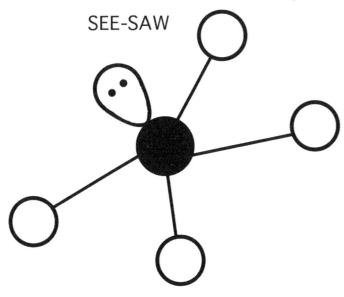

ATOMIC STRUCTURE: Geometric Family

T - SHAPED

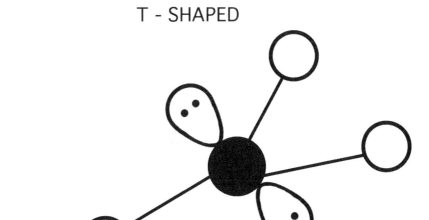

ATOMIC STRUCTURE: Geometric Family

TRIGONAL PLANAR

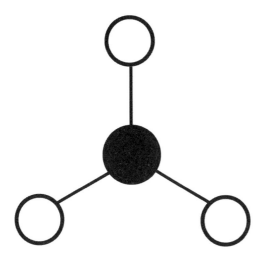

ATOMIC STRUCTURE: Geometric Family

SQUARE PRYAMID

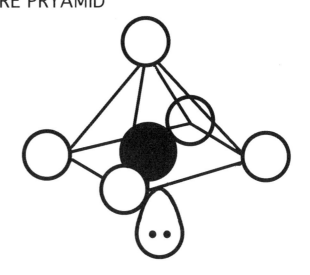

ATOMIC STRUCTURE: Geometric Family

TRIGONAL PYRAMID

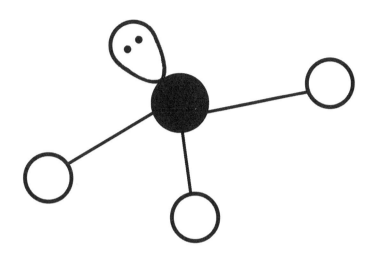

BONDING: Nomenclature

Monoatomic Negative Ions

H^- hydride N^{-3} nitride O^{-2} oxide F^- fluoride
P^{-3} phosphide S^{-2} sulfide Cl^- chloride Br^- bromide

Transition Metals with one or more positive ions

Fe^{+2} ferrous Fe^{+3} ferric Cu^+ cuprous Cu^{+2} cupric
Mn^{+2} manganous Mn^{+3} manganic Sn^{+2} stannous Sn^{+4} stannic

Common Acids and Bases

HCl^- hydrochloric H^2SO^4 sulfuric HNO^3 nitric
H^3PO^4 phosphoric H^2CO^{-3} carbonic   NaOH sodium hydroxide
NH^4OH ammonium hydroxide

ATOMIC STRUCTURE: Geometric Family

TETRAHEDRAL

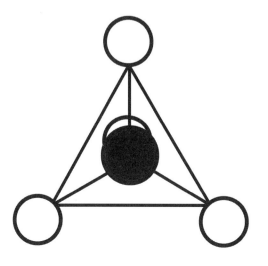

BONDING: Chemical Formulas

CHEMICAL FORMULA: represents the molar composition of a molecule.

MOLECULAR FORMULA: represents the makeup of a molecule of any
   given substance. Molecular formula accurately conveys the
   number of atoms of each element needed to form a molecule
   (ex: NaCl).

EMPIRICAL FORMULA: represents the simplest ratio in which atoms
   can bind to each other to form a specific compound.
Example: H_2O_2 (molecular formula of hydrogen peroxide)
HO (empirical formula of hydrogen peroxide)

• When molecular formulas of ionic substances are written, the metal
   ion is written first followed by the non-metal ion.
• When molecular formulas of covalent substances are written, the
   nonmetal with the lowest electronegativity is written first
   followed by the rest in increasing order.

BONDING: Types

NONPOLAR COVALENT BOND: is formed between two atoms with identical electronegativity. As a result, the bonding electrons are equally shared by the two atoms (ex: O_2 or Cl_2).

POLAR COVALENT BOND: is formed between two atoms of varying electronegativity. In polar covalent bond, the bonding electrons tend to spend more time around the atom with higher electronegativity. As a result, there is a nonsymmetrical charge distribution in the bond leading to a partial negative and positive ends in the molecule (ex: $+H_2O^-$).

COORDINATE COVALENT BOND: is formed when the pair of electrons shared in the bond is contributed by one of the two atoms (ex: NH_4^+).

METALLIC BOND: is formed between metals. Since metallic ions cannot assume the electron configuration of inert gases by donating or sharing electrons, it is impossible for two metals to bind to each other via ionic or covalent bond.

BONDING: Types of Bonds

CHEMICAL BONDS: occur when two atomic nuclei share or transfer electrons between them. When a chemical bond is formed, energy is released. On the other hand, energy is required to break bonds. The strength of a chemical bond depends on the amount of energy released at the time of its formation. The greater the amount of energy released, the stronger the bond and vice versa.

TWO MAJOR TYPES OF BONDS
- **IONIC BONDS:** are formed when a metal reacts with a non-metal. Ionic bonds are characterized by the fact that electron(s) from the metallic nuclei are transferred to nuclei of the non-metals. The complete transfer of electrons produce charged particles called ions.
- **COVALENT BONDS:** are formed between two non-metals. Unlike ionic bonds, there are no transfer of electron(s) in covalent bonds. Rather the two non-metals equally or unequally share electrons between them. When electrons are equally shared by the non-metals the bond is termed as non-polar covalent. And when they are unequally shared, the bond is known as polar covalent.

GAS LAWS: Charles' Law

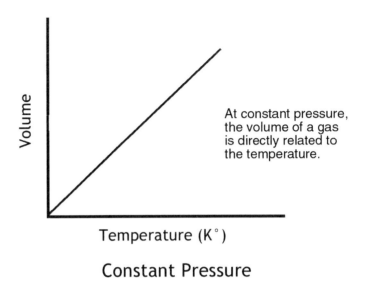

At constant pressure, the volume of a gas is directly related to the temperature.

Constant Pressure

CATALYSTS

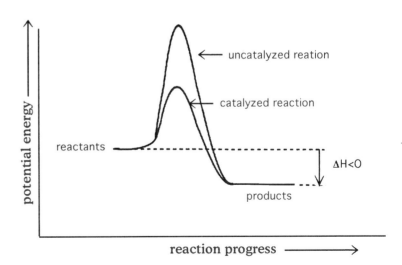

DISPERSION FORCE

INSTANTANEOUS DIPOLE   INSTANTANEOUS DIPOLE

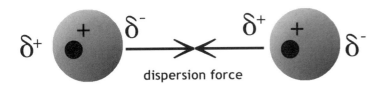

ELECTROCHEMISTRY: Galvanic Cell

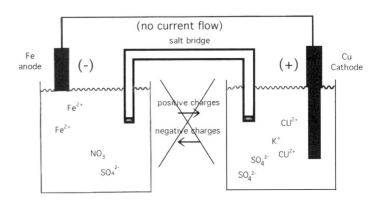

Current flow ceases when the anode is consumed.
REDOX reaction is no longer possible.

COULOMB'S LAW

Q_1 = change of particle #1 (in coulombs)

Q_2 = change of particle #2 (in coulombs)

k = Coulomb's Constant

$= 9.0 \times 10^9\, \text{N-m}^2/\text{C}^2$

Force of electrostatic → $F = k\dfrac{Q_1 \times Q_2}{R_2}$
interaction (in Newtons)

R_2 = distance between the charges (in meters)

ELECTROLYTIC CELLS

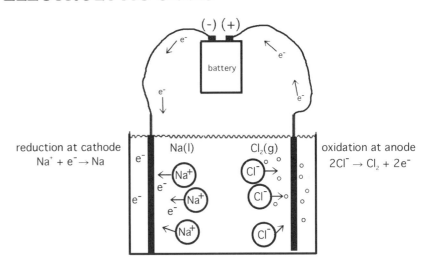

reduction at cathode
$Na^+ + e^- \rightarrow Na$

oxidation at anode
$2Cl^- \rightarrow Cl_2 + 2e^-$

Electrolytic cell requires infusion of electrons from an external battery to work.

ELECTROCHEMISTRY: Galvanic Cells

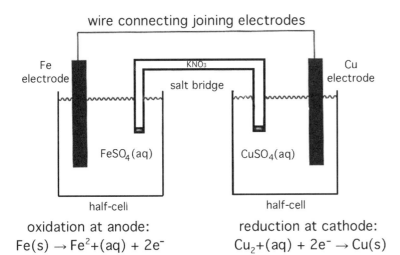

oxidation at anode:
$$Fe(s) \rightarrow Fe^{2}+(aq) + 2e^-$$

reduction at cathode:
$$Cu_2+(aq) + 2e^- \rightarrow Cu(s)$$

ELECTROCHEMISTRY: Galvanic Cell

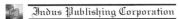
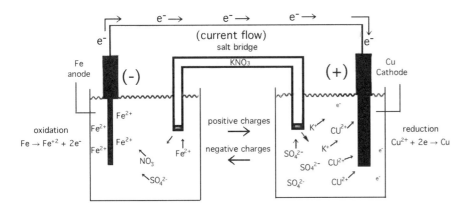

Galvanic cells generate current through spontaneous REDOX reactions. No external batteries are required.

EQUILIBRIUM ENERGY: K_{eq} And Gibb's Free Energy

$$\Delta G = \Delta H - T\Delta S$$
$$A + B \rightarrow C + D$$

$\triangle G$ = -2.3 RT log Keq (where $\triangle G$ = Gibbs Free Energy, R = Universal Gas Constant, T = temperature in °K)

• The negative value of $\triangle G$ indicates that the reaction in the forward direction is spontaneous. A positive and high Keq constant also indicated a spontaneous forward reaction.

• The total change in equilibrium in free energy is zero.

ELECTRONEGATIVITY TREND
(The Periodic Table)

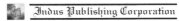
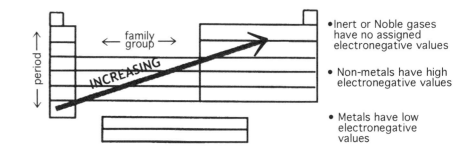

• Inert or Noble gases have no assigned electronegative values

• Non-metals have high electronegative values

• Metals have low electronegative values

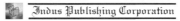
EQUILIBRIUM: Le Chatelier's Principle

LE CHATELIER'S PRINCIPLE: states that change in concentration, pressure, and temperature affect the equilibrium state of a chemical system.

CONCENTRATION $A + B \longrightarrow C + D$
1. Increase in concentration of any one of the reactants favors the forward reaction.
2. Addition of products favors the reverse reaction.
3. Removal of product(s) favor the forward reaction.

TEMPERATURE
1. Increase in temperature favors endothermic reactions $A + B + heat \longrightarrow C + D$
2. Decrease in temperature favors exothermic reactions $A + B \longrightarrow C + D + heat$

PRESSURE: (only affects reactants or products that are in the gaseous phase)
1. Increase in pressure shifts a reaction from the side with the higher moles of gas(es) to the side with the lower moles of gas(es). ↑Pressure + ↑Pressure + $N_2 + 3H_2 \longrightarrow 2NH_3$
2. Decrease in pressure shifts a reaction from the side with the lower moles of gas(es) to the side with the higher moles of gas(es). ↓Pressure + $N_2 + 3H_2 \longleftarrow 2NH_3$

ENERGY LEVELS

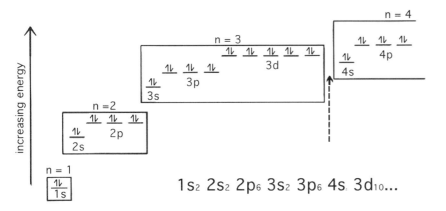

$1s_2 \; 2s_2 \; 2p_6 \; 3s_2 \; 3p_6 \; 4s \; 3d_{10}...$

GEBERAL ORDER OF FILLING

$$1s_2 \; 2s_2 \; 2p_6 \; 3s_2 \; 3p_6 \; 4s_2 \; 3d_{10}...$$

[Memorize This!]

GAS PHASE: Phases of Matter

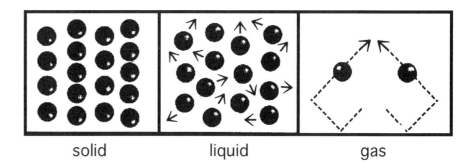

solid   liquid   gas

FLUIDS: Heat Formula

TEMPERATURE CHANGE IN FLUIDS

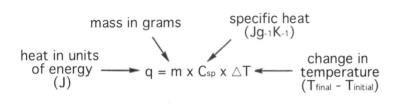

mass in grams

specific heat
$(Jg^{-1}K^{-1})$

heat in units
of energy
(J) → $q = m \times C_{sp} \times \triangle T$ ← change in
temperature
$(T_{final} - T_{initial})$

ENERGY LEVELS: Hydrogen Atom

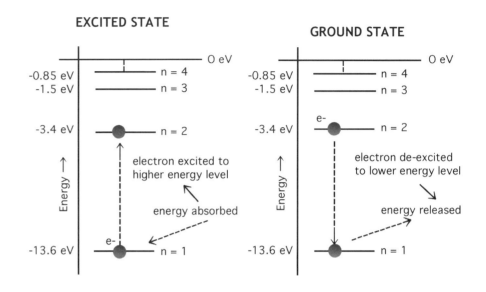

EXCITED STATE

0 eV

-0.85 eV — n = 4
-1.5 eV — n = 3

-3.4 eV — n = 2

electron excited to
higher energy level

energy absorbed

Energy →

-13.6 eV e- — n = 1

GROUND STATE

0 eV

-0.85 eV — n = 4
-1.5 eV — n = 3

-3.4 eV e- — n = 2

electron de-excited
to lower energy level

energy released

Energy →

-13.6 eV — n = 1

PHASES OF MATTER: Sublimation

DIRECT CHANGE OF PHASE FROM SOLID TO GAS

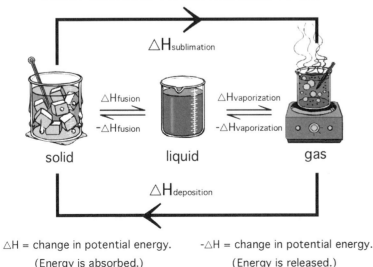

$\triangle H_{sublimation}$

$\triangle H_{fusion}$

$-\triangle H_{fusion}$

$\triangle H_{vaporization}$

$-\triangle H_{vaporization}$

solid   liquid   gas

$\triangle H_{deposition}$

$\triangle H$ = change in potential energy.
(Energy is absorbed.)

$-\triangle H$ = change in potential energy.
(Energy is released.)

HEAT FORMULA: Change Of Phase
(constant temperature)

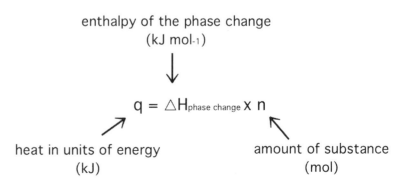

enthalpy of the phase change
$(kJ \ mol^{-1})$

↓

$q = \triangle H_{phase\ change} \times n$

heat in units of energy
(kJ)

amount of substance
(mol)

THE PERIODIC TABLE: Atom Size

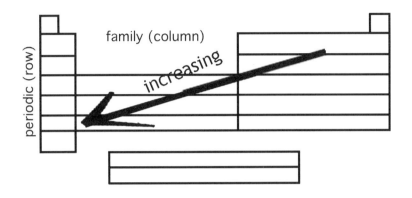

MOLECULAR PROPERTIES: Common Lewis Acids

$$H_2O \quad HBr \quad HCl \quad H_2SO_4 \quad HNO_3 \quad LI^+ \quad Mg^{+2} \quad Br^+$$

OH
Phenol

$CH_3CH_2CH_2OH$
alcohol

$$R - \overset{\overset{\displaystyle O}{\|}}{C} - OH$$
carboxylic
acid

GAS LAWS: The Ideal Gas Law

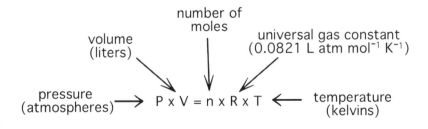

Gases behave ideally in high temperature and low pressure.

MOLECULAR PROPERTIES

$$\textbf{FORMAL CHARGE} = \begin{pmatrix} \text{\# of} \\ \text{valence electrons} \\ \text{in free atom} \end{pmatrix} - \begin{pmatrix} \text{\# of} \\ \text{Valence electrons} \\ \text{in bound atom} \end{pmatrix}$$

$$= \begin{pmatrix} \text{\# of} \\ \text{valence} \\ \text{electrons} \end{pmatrix} - \begin{pmatrix} \text{\# of} \\ \text{non-bonding} \\ \text{elecrtons} \end{pmatrix} - \begin{pmatrix} \text{half of} \\ \text{bonding} \\ \text{electrons} \end{pmatrix}$$

SIMPLE TESTS: Common Tests and Reactions

TEST	SIGNIFANCE
BLOOD UREA NITROGEN (BUN)	Used to assess kidney function
HUMAN CHORIONIC GONADOTROPIN	Determination of pregnancy
CREATINE CLEARANCE	Used to assess renal functions
GLUCOSE TOLERANCE TEST	To detect hyperglycemia *(diabetes mellinus)*
TOLLENS' TEST - AG$^+$ in NH$_3$(aq)	Positive results identify aldehydes
BENEDICT'S REGENT	Positive results identify oxidation of monosaccharides
FEHLING'S REGENT	Positive results identify oxidation of monosaccharides
KILIANI-FISCHER SYNTHESIS	Increases the chain length of monosaccharides
WOHL DEGRADATION	Decreases the chain length of monosaccharides

THE PERIODIC TABLE: Trends

ATOMIC NUMBER: is the number of protons in the nucleus of an element.
MASS NUMBER: is the number of protons plus neutrons in the nucleus of an element.

TRENDS IN THE PERIODIC TABLE
- **# OF PROTONS:** As the atomic # increases, the number of protons in elements also increases.
- **# OF VALENCE ELECTRONS:** As the atomic # increases, the # of valence electrons in an atom increases as well.
- **IONIZATION ENERGY:** As the atomic # increases, the ionization energy also increases.
- **ELECTRONEGATIVITY:** As the atomic # increases, the electronegativity also increases.

TRENDS IN A GROUP
- **# OF VALENCE ELECTRONS:** As the atomic # increases, the # of valence electrons in an atom remains the same.
- **IONIZATION ENERGY:** As the atomic # increases, the ionization energy decreases.
- **ELECTRONEGATIVITY:** As the atomic # increases, the electronegativity decreases.

Colligative Properties: Osmotic Pressure

semipermeable membrane
(only permeable to water)

water

solute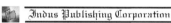

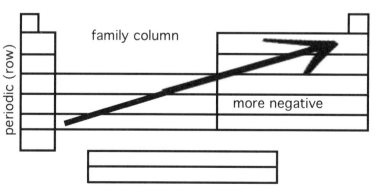

← direction of osmosis

THE PERIODIC TABLE: Electron Affinity

Noble gases are expected from this trend

family column

periodic (row)

more negative

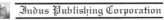

PHASES OF MATTER: Gas Formula

IDEAL GAS LAW: expresses the combined relationship between the pressure, volume and temperature of a gas as defined by Boyle, Charles, and Gay-Lussac.

$$\frac{P_1 V_1}{T_1} = \frac{P_2 V_2}{T_2} = nR$$

P = pressure in atm
T = temperature in °K
V = volume, n = moles of the gas
R = universal gas constant (0.821 atm)

• L/mole• °K)

$$PV = nRT$$

GRAHAM'S LAW: states that the rate of diffusion of gases is inversely proportional to the square root of its molecular weight.
$$v_1 / v_2 = \sqrt{m_2 / m_1}$$ v = velocity and m = molecular weight of the gas

PARTIAL PRESSURE: of a gas in a mixture is proportional to its mole ratio in the mixture.

Pgas A = moles of gas A / total moles of all gases in the mixture

---

PHASES OF MATTER: Phase Change Curve

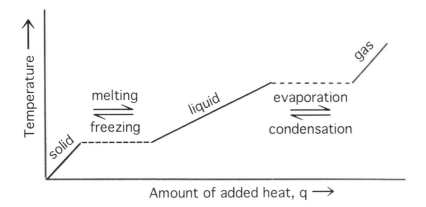

NOTE: Temperature remains constant during phase changes.

PHASES OF MATTER

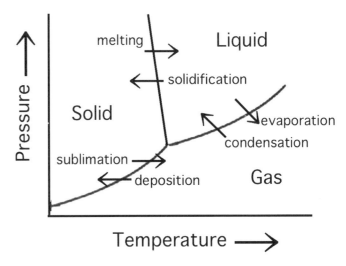

NOTE: The negative slope between the solid and liquid phases.

PHASES OF MATTER: Gases

Standard Temperature and Pressure (STP)

The STP is defined as the state of the environment when the pressure is equal to 760 mm Hg (torr) or 1 atm and the temperature is 0°C (273°K).

Gas Moles and Molar Volume

One mole of any gas = 22.4 liters = 6.02×10^{23} particles (Avogadro's number)

Kinetic Theory of Gases

1. There are no forces of attraction between gas molecules.
2. When gas molecules collide, energy may be transferred between molecules. However, the net energy of the system remains constant.
3. The volume of all gas molecules when combined is negligible in comparison to the volume of space they occupy.
4. All gas molecules move in a random fashion.

PHASES OF MATTER: Liquids

LIQUID MOLECULES are not arranged in any order. Like gas molecules, liquid molecules are in constant motion. However, attractive forces exists between neighboring liquid molecules (ex: H-bond in water). While liquids do not have a defined shape, they have definite volume.

HEAT OF FUSION: is the amount of energy required to melt a unit mass of a solid to liquid.

HEAT OF VAPORIZATION: is the amount of energy required to vaporize a unit mass of liquid to gas.

FREEZING POINT: is the temperature at which a given liquid freezes to become a solid.

BOILING POINT: is the temperature at which a given liquid vaporizes to become a gas.

BOILING POINT & VAPOR PRESSURE: At boiling point, the vapor pressure (the pressure exerted by liquid molecules escaping into gaseous phase) must EQUAL the atmospheric pressure.

PHASES OF MATTER: Gases

Under ideal conditions (low pressure and high temperature), gases behave in a predictable manner. Based on their behavior, the pressure, volume, and temperature of gases can be quantified.

BOYLE'S LAW: states that if the temperature remains constant, the pressure and the volume of a gas varies inversely with each other.

$$P_1 V_1 = P_2 V_2$$

(P_1, V_1 = initial pressure & volume)
(P_2, V_2 = new pressure & volume)

CHARLES'S LAW: states that if the pressure remains constant, the temperature and the volume of a gas varies directly with each other.

$$T_2 V_1 = T_1 V_2$$

(T_1, V_1 = initial temperature & volume)
(T_2, V_2 = new temperature & volume)

GENERAL SHAPE OF AN S ORBITAL

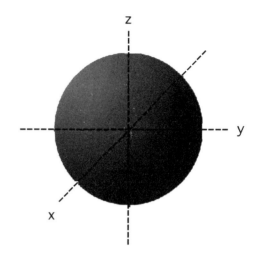

PHASES OF MATTER: Solids

SOLIDS are characterized by ordered molecular structures, definite shapes and volumes.

Because of the nature of solids, they are chemically inert relative to liquids and gases.

MELTING POINT: is the temperature at which a specific solid melts to form its corresponding liquid (ex: ice to water). At melting point, the kinetic energy of the particles that compose a solid is high enough to overcome the attractive forces that exist between particles. Melting cannot take place unless intermolecular attractive forces are broken.

SUBLIMATION: is the process in which a solid directly vaporizes to gas without going through the transitory liquid phase.

SOLUTION: Characteristics Of Mixtures vs. Compounds

COMPARISONS OF GENERAL CHARACTERISTICS

MIXTURES

1. Can be separated by physical means only

2. Elements form no definite proportions

3. Mixtures are formed by physical unions

4. Mixtures preserve the chemical identity of each compound

COMPOUND

1. Can be separated by chemical reactions only

2. Compounds are formed of definite proportions of elements

3. Compounds are formed via chemical reactions.

4. Each compound represents an unique substance

SOLUTION: Colligative Properties

COLLIGATIVE PROPERTIES: are based on the scientific fact that dissolved particles (solute) affect some of the physical properties of a solvent. The properties that are affected are: the boiling point, freezing point, osmotic pressure, and vapor pressure.

Boiling Point Elevation = Kbmn (Kb=boiling point constant of a specific solvent) (m=molality, n=# of particles)

Freezing Point Depression = Kfmn (Kf=freezing point constant of a specific solvent) (m=molality, n=# of particles)

Osmotic Pressure = pV = nRT   (p=osmotic pressure, V=volume, T=temperature) (n=moles of solute, R=universal gas constant)

Vapor Pressure = The vapor pressure and the boiling point of a solution is directly related to each other. Both of them increase or decrease simultaneously.

TABLE OF REACTION SPONTANEITY

$\triangle H_{rxn}$	$\triangle S_{rxn}$	$\triangle G_{rxn}$	
−	+	−	Spontaneous
0	+	−	
−	0	−	
+	−	+	Not Spontaneous
0	−	+	
+	0	+	
+	+*	+ or −	Depends On Relative Magnitude of △H
−	−	+ or −	and T△S
$T\triangle S_{rxn}$	$T\triangle S_{rxn}$	0	At Equilibrium

* Reactions with △S > 0 always become spontaneous at suffucuently high temperature.

SOLUTION: Concentration Units

MOLARITY (M) = moles/L   or (grams/molecular weight)/liters

MOLALITY = moles of solute/kilograms of solvent = moles/Kg

MOLES OF SOLUTE = molarity X volume

GRAMS OF SOLUTE = moles of solute X mole mass of solute

EQUIVALENTS = grams/equivalent weight

NORMALITY = equivalents of solute/liters of solution

THE OCTET

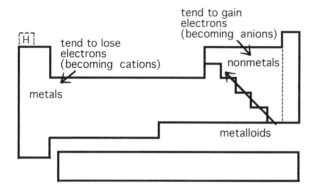

THERMODYNAMICS: Measurement of Energy

The unit of measurement of energy in chemical reactions is calories or kilocalories (kcal).

FOR WATER: # of calories = grams of water $X \triangle T$ (T=temperature)

FOR ALL OTHER OBJECTS: # of calories X specific heat of the object

$$(c) \; X \; \triangle T$$

TEMPERATURE CONVERSION

$$°F = (9/5)(C°) + 32 \quad and \quad K = (°C) + 273.15$$

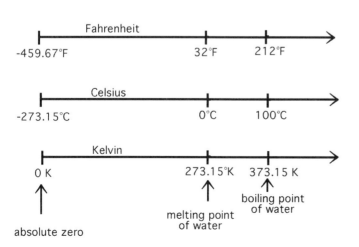

THERMODYNAMICS: Reactions

During all chemical reactions, energy is either released or absorbed. Energy is absorbed when chemical bonds are broken. On the other hand, energy is released when new bonds are formed.

EXOTHERMIC REACTIONS: All reactions that release heat (or energy) when products are formed are defined as exothermic reactions. In exothermic reactions, the reactants have higher potential energy than the products.

ENDOTHERMIC REACTIONS: All reactions that absorb heat (or energy) when products are formed are defined as endothermic reactions. In endothermic reactions, the reactants have lower potential energy than the products.

ACTIVATION ENERGY: is the minimum amount of energy required to start a reaction. Usually, exothermic reactions have low activation energy while endothermic reactions display high activation energy.

THERMODYNAMICS: Laws

FIRST LAW OF THERMODYNAMICS: states that energy can be neither created nor destroyed.

SECOND LAW OF THERMODYNAMICS: states that energy (heat) is transferred unidirectionally from an area of high temperature to an area of low temperature.

THIRD LAW OF THERMODYNAMICS: At absolute zero (temperature), the entropy of all pure solids is said to be zero.

VAPOR PRESSURE

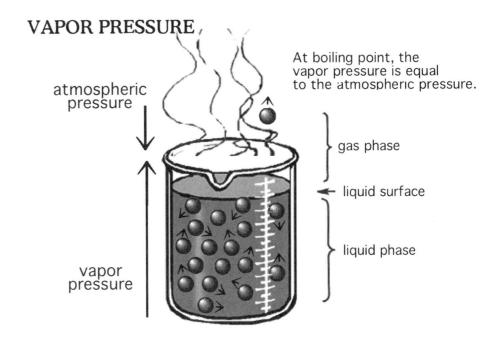

At boiling point, the vapor pressure is equal to the atmospheric pressure.

atmospheric pressure

gas phase

liquid surface

vapor pressure

liquid phase

THERMODYNAMICS: Types Of Energy

ENERGY

ENERGY is defined as an object's capacity to do work. Energy cannot be created or destroyed.

- **KINETIC ENERGY:** is the energy associated with objects when they are in motion.
- **POTENTIAL ENERGY:** is an object's "stored" energy. An object's ability to do work is directly proportional to its potential energy.
- **HEAT:** is the energy associated with the temperature of an object. When the temperature varies, heat is either released or absorbed by an object/system.
- **CHEMICAL ENERGY:** is the amount of energy that is absorbed or released during chemical reactions.
- **ELECTRICAL ENERGY:** is defined as the energy generated as a result of electrical current.
- **NUCLEAR ENERGY:** is associated with changes in the mass of atoms.
- **LIGHT:** is the energy associated with the electromagnetic waves.

THERMODYNAMICS: Entropy

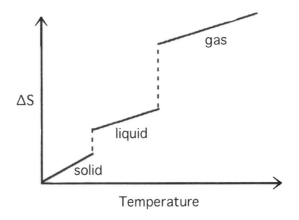

gas

ΔS

liquid

solid

Temperature

Gases have the highest entropy because of greater randomness

ACID DERIVATIVE & REACTIVITY

ACID DERIVATIVE	LEAVING GROUP
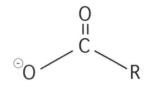	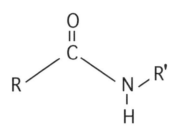
acid anhydride	conjugate base of a weak acidic acid

ACID DERIVATIVE & REACTIVITY

Acid Derivative	Leaving Group

Amide	Conjugate base of an amine (poor leaving group)

ACID DERIVATIVE & REACTIVITY

ACID DERIVATIVE	LEAVING GROUP
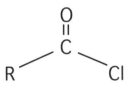	Cl^-
acid chloride	chlorine ion (good leaving group)

ACID DERIVATIVE & REACTIVITY

Acid Derivative	Leaving Group
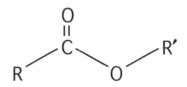	
Ester	An alkoxide ion (poor leaving group)

ALKENES: The Markovnikoff Rule

The rule states that in an addition reaction, H is added to the <u>least</u> substituted carbon in a double bond:

MARKOVNIKOFF REACTION:

$$H_3C-CH=CH_2 + HCl \longrightarrow H_3C-\overset{\overset{\displaystyle H}{\displaystyle |}}{\underset{\underset{\displaystyle Cl}{\displaystyle |}}{C}}-CH_3$$

ANTI - MARKOVNIKOFF REACTION:

$$H_3C-CH=CH_2 + HCl \longrightarrow H_3C-CH_2-CH_2Cl$$

ACID DERIVATIVES:

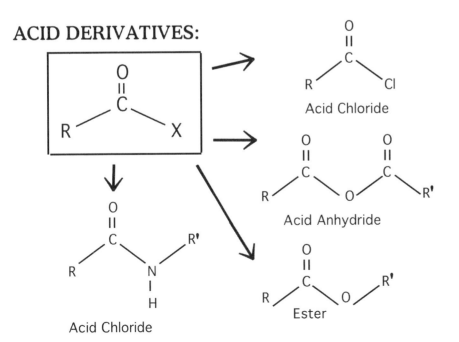

Acid Chloride

Acid Anhydride

Ester

Acid Chloride

SUBSTITUTED AROMATIC RINGS

META-DIRECTING DEACTIVATORS

- NO_2	- $CO_2CH_2CH_3$
- COOH	- $COCH_3$
- CN	- $COCH_3$
-CHO	- $N(CH_3)_3$

COMMON APROTIC SOLVENTS

1) Hexane

2) Diethyl Ether

3) Dimethyl Sulfoxide (DMSO)

4) Chloroform

5) Benzene

BENT

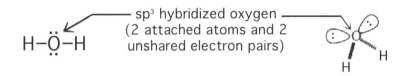

sp³ hybridized oxygen
(2 attached atoms and 2
unshared electron pairs)

CONJUGATE ACIDS & BASES

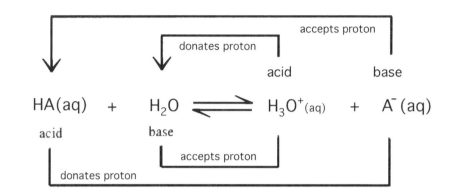

accepts proton

donates proton

acid   base

$$HA(aq) \;+\; H_2O \;\rightleftharpoons\; H_3O^+{}_{(aq)} \;+\; A^-(aq)$$

acid   base

accepts proton

donates proton

BENZENE DERIVATIVES

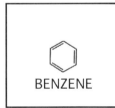

BENZENE

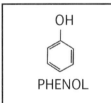

OH

PHENOL

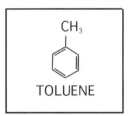

CH₃

TOLUENE

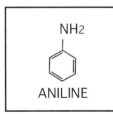

NH2

ANILINE

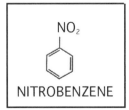

NO₂

NITROBENZENE

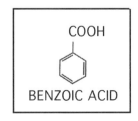

COOH

BENZOIC ACID

COMMON REACTIONS: Carboxylic Acids

ACID HALIDES

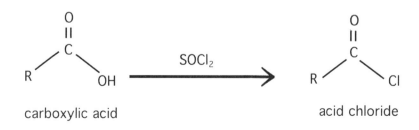

carboxylic acid $SOCl_2$ acid chloride

DEHYDRATION OF ALCOHOLS

tert - butyl alcohol   isobutylene

NOTE: look for an acid and change in temperature in dehydration rxn.

SUBSTITUENT EFFECTS

[ELECTROPHILIC AROMATIC SUBSTITUTION]

SUBSTITUENT	INDUCTIVE EFFECT	RESONANCE EFFECT
- $\ddot{O}H$	electron withdrawing	electron donating
- $\ddot{N}H^2$	electron withdrawing	electron donating
-F, -Cl, -Br, -I	electron withdrawing	electron donating
-CH_3	electron donating	————————

CYCLOHEXANE

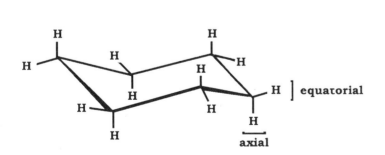

equatorial

axial

DIASTEREOMERS:

... NON-SUPERIMPOSABLE, NON-MIRROR IMAGES

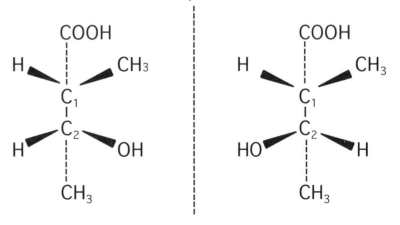

All diastereomers must have at least 2 chiral carbons.

FUNCTIONAL GROUP: Acetal

ACETAL

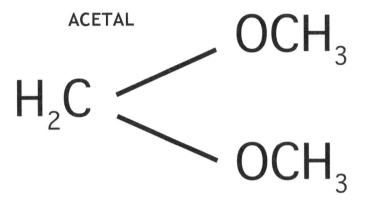

FUNCTIONAL GROUP: Acid Halide

ACID HALIDE

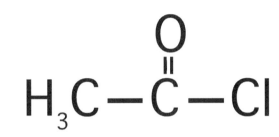

ENANTIOMERS:

NON-SUPERIMPOSABLE MIRROR IMAGES

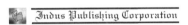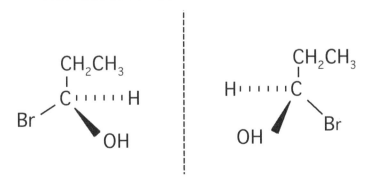

Mirror Plane

FUNCTIONAL GROUP: Acid Anhydride

ANHYDRIDE

FUNCTIONAL GROUP: Aldehyde

ALDEHYDE

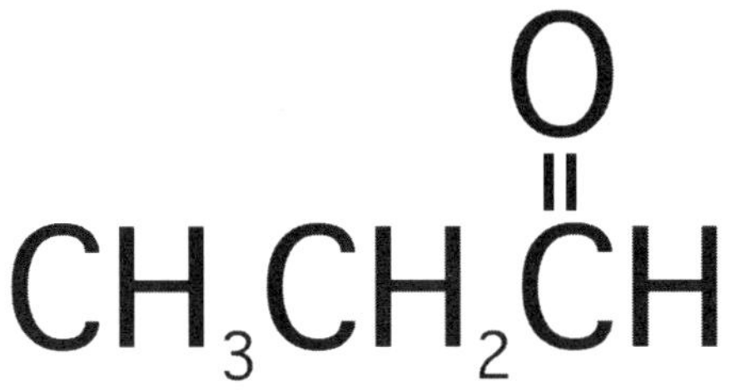

$$CH_3CH_2\overset{\overset{\displaystyle O}{\|}}{C}H$$

ORGANIC STRUCTURE: Alkene

ALKENE
(Double Bond)

$$H_2C=CH_2$$

FUNCTIONAL GROUP: Alcohol

ALCOHOL

$$CH_3CH_2CH_2OH$$

ORGANIC STRUCTURE: Alkane

ALKANE
(Single Bond)

$$H_3C-CH_3$$

FUNCTIONAL GROUP: Amide

AMIDE

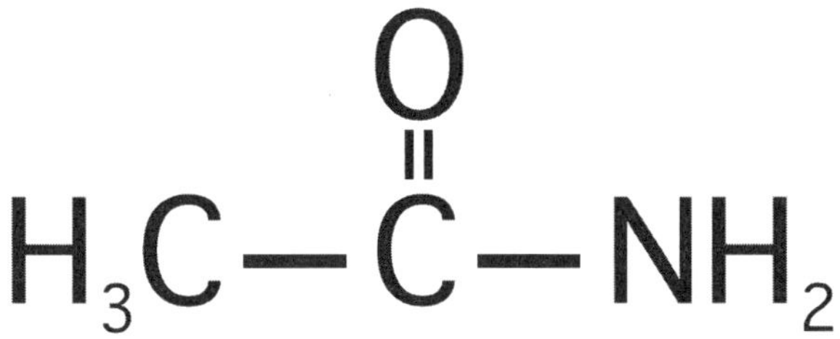

$$H_3C - \overset{\overset{\displaystyle O}{\|}}{C} - NH_2$$

FUNCTIONAL GROUP: Carboxylic Acid

Carboxylic Acid

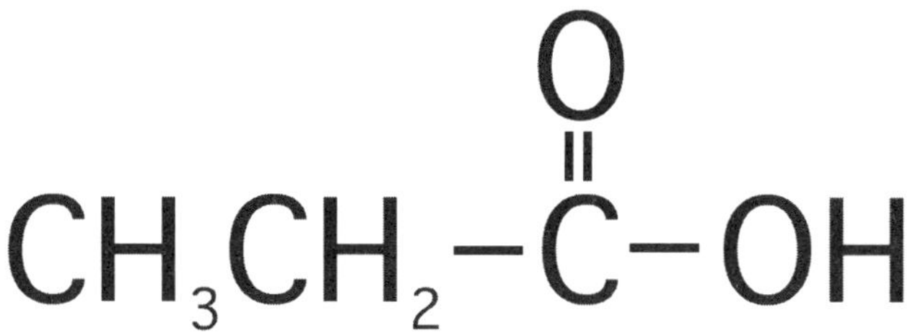

$$CH_3CH_2 - \overset{\overset{\displaystyle O}{\|}}{C} - OH$$

ORGANIC STRUCTURE: Alkyne

ALKYNE
(Triple Bond)

$$HC \equiv CH$$

FUNCTIONAL GROUP: Amine

Amine

$$H_3C - CH_2NH_2$$

FUNCTIONAL GROUP: Ester

ESTER

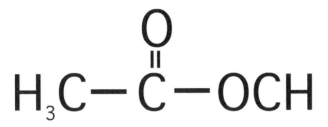

$$H_3C-\overset{\overset{\displaystyle O}{\|}}{C}-OCH$$

FUNCTIONAL GROUP: Acid Hemiacetal

HEMIACETAL

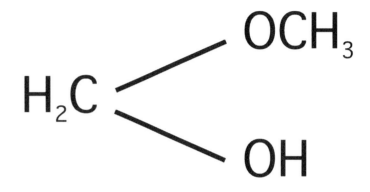

$$H_2C \overset{\displaystyle OCH_3}{\underset{\displaystyle OH}{<}}$$

FUNCTIONAL GROUP: Epoxide

EPOXIDE

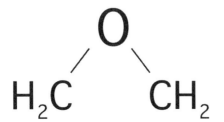

$$H_2C \overset{\displaystyle O}{\diagup \diagdown} CH_2$$

FUNCTIONAL GROUP: Ether

ETHER

$$CH_3CH_2-O-CH_2CH_3$$

FUNCTIONAL GROUP: Phenol

PHENOL

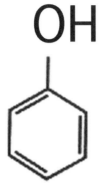

OH

MOLECULAR PROPERTIES

COMMON LEWIS BASES: look for a carbonyl carbon

ALCOHOL: $CH_3\ddot{C}H_2OH$	**ETHER**

$$\begin{array}{c} :O: \\ \parallel \end{array}$$
ALDEHYDE: CH_3CH **ACID CHLORIDE**

$$\begin{array}{c} :O: \\ \parallel \end{array}$$
KETONE: CH_3CCH_3 **ESTER**

$$\begin{array}{c} :O: \\ \parallel .. \end{array}$$
CARBOXYLIC ACID: $CH_3\ddot{C}OH$ **AMINE**

FUNCTIONAL GROUP: Ketone

KETONE

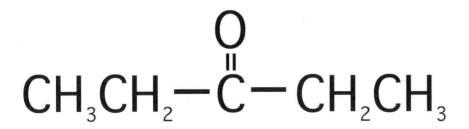

$$CH_3CH_2-\overset{\overset{\textstyle O}{\parallel}}{C}-CH_2CH_3$$

THE GRIGNARD REGENT

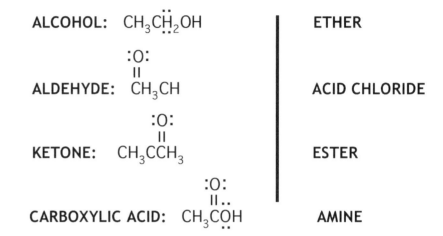

1) $RMgBr + H\overset{\overset{\textstyle O}{\parallel}}{C}H \longrightarrow R-CH_2OMgBr \xrightarrow{H^+} RCH_2OH$ (primary alcohol)

2) $RMgBr + R_1CHO \xrightarrow{ether} R-\overset{\overset{\textstyle R_1}{|}}{\underset{\underset{\textstyle H}{|}}{C}}-OH$ (secondary alcohol)

3) $RMgBr + R_1-\overset{\overset{\textstyle R_2}{|}}{C}=O \xrightarrow{ether} R_1-\overset{\overset{\textstyle R_2}{|}}{\underset{\underset{\textstyle R_1}{|}}{C}}-OH$ (tertiary alcohol)

ORBITALS: 3 p Orbitals

THE 3 p ORBITALS

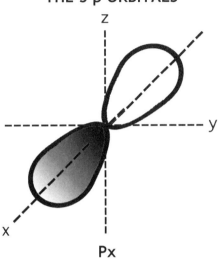

Px

ORBITALS: 3 p Orbitals

THE 3 p ORBITALS

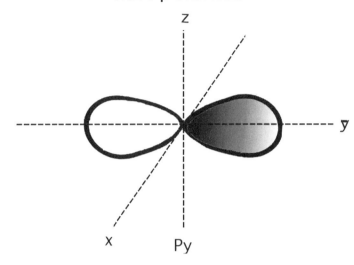

Py

MOLECULAR PROPERTIES

Stereochemistry - Cyclohexane Conformations

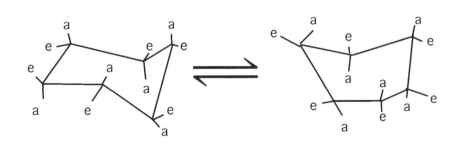

a = axial position   e = equational position

ORBITALS: 3 p Orbitals

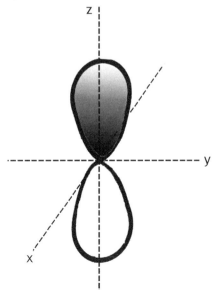

ORBITLAS: 5 p Orbitals

THE 5 p ORBITALS

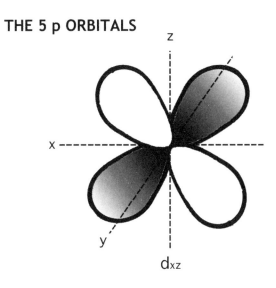

d_{xz}

ORBITALS: 5 p Orbitals

THE 5 p ORBITAL

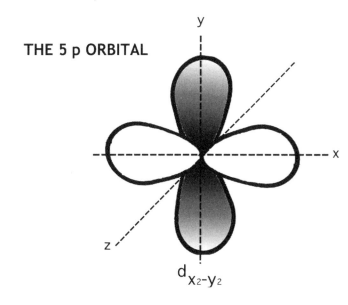

$d_{x_2-y_2}$

ORBITLAS: 5 p Orbitals

THE 5 p ORBITALS

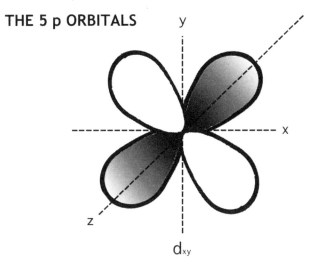

d_{xy}

ORBITALS: 5 p Orbitals

THE 5 p ORBITAL

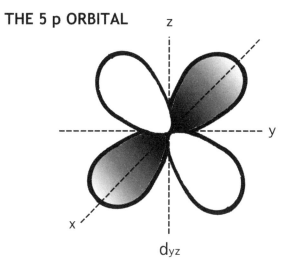

d_{yz}

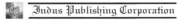
THE ORDER OF REACTIVITY

(NUCLEOPHITIC SUBSTITUTION REACTIONS)

Acid Chlorides > Acid Anhydrides > Esters > Amides

ORGANIC STRUCTURE: Common Name

ORGANIC STRUCTURE	COMMON NAME	IUPAC NAME
$R-CH_2CH_2CH_2CH_3$	n - Butyl	Butyl
$R-\underset{\underset{CH_3}{\vert}}{C}HCH_2CH_3$	sec - Butyl	1 - methyl propyl
$R-CH_2\underset{\underset{CH_3}{\vert}}{C}HCH_3$	Isobutyl	2- methyl propyl
$R-\overset{\overset{CH_3}{\vert}}{\underset{\underset{CH_3}{\vert}}{C}}-CH_3$	tert - Butyl	1,1 - Dimethyl ethyl

 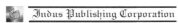
ORBITALS: 5 p Orbitals

THE 5 p ORBITALS

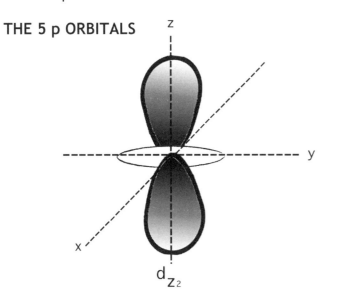

d_{z^2}

SUMMARY OF ORGANIC REACTION TYPES

ADDITION: $A + B \longrightarrow C$

ELIMINATION: $A \longrightarrow B + C$

SUBSTITUTION: $A - B + C - D \rightarrow A - D + B - C$

REARRANGEMENT: $A \longrightarrow B$

OXIDATION & REDUCTION REACTIONS

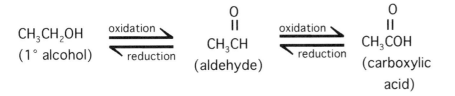

$$CH_3CH_2OH \xrightarrow[\text{reduction}]{\text{oxidation}} CH_3CH \xrightarrow[\text{reduction}]{\text{oxidation}} CH_3COH$$

(1° alcohol) (aldehyde) (carboxylic acid)

$$CH_3CHOH \xrightarrow[\text{reduction}]{\text{oxidation}} CH_3CCH_3$$

(2° alcohol) (ketone)

OXIDATION & REDUCTION
OF ORGANIC COMPOUNDS

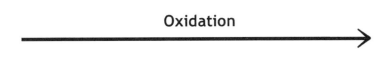

Oxidation

Alcohol   Aldehyde / Ketone   Carboxylic Acid

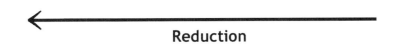

Reduction

COMMON PROTIC SOLVENTS

1) Water

2) Ethanol

3) Acetic Acid

4) Methanol

PRIMARY, SECONDARY & TERTIARY
ALCOHOLS

$$HO - \underset{\underset{H}{|}}{\overset{\overset{H}{|}}{C}} - CH_2CH_3 \qquad HO - \underset{\underset{CH_3}{|}}{\overset{\overset{H}{|}}{C}} - CH_2CH_3 \qquad OH - \underset{\underset{CH_3}{|}}{\overset{\overset{CH_3}{|}}{C}} - CH_2CH_3$$

PRIMARY (1°)   SECONDARY (2°)   TERTIARY (3°)

[2 Hydrogens]   [1 Hydrogen]   [No Hydrogens]

COMMON REACTION: Aldehyde and/or Ketone

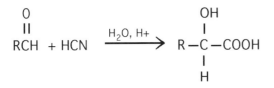

$$RCH + HCN \xrightarrow{H_2O,\ H+} R-\overset{OH}{\underset{H}{C}}-COOH$$

$$RCH + NaHSO_3 \longrightarrow R-\overset{OH}{\underset{H}{C}}-SO_3^- Na^+$$

COMMON REACTIONS: Carboxylic Acids

ESTERS

$$R-\overset{O}{\overset{||}{C}}-OH + R_1OH \longrightarrow R_1-\overset{O}{\overset{||}{C}}-OR + H_2O$$

carboxylic acid   Alcohol   Ester

PYRAMIDAL SHAPES

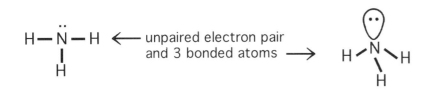

← unpaired electron pair and 3 bonded atoms →

COMMON REACTIONS: Carboxylic Acids

ANHYDRIDE

carboxylic acid   +   carboxylic acid   →   Anhydride

+H_2O

REACTIVITY OF ALKYL HALIDES

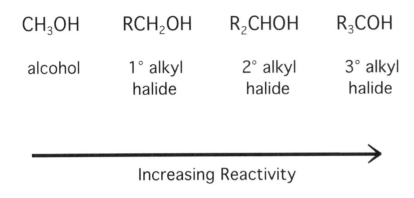

CH_3OH RCH_2OH R_2CHOH R_3COH

alcohol   1° alkyl halide   2° alkyl halide   3° alkyl halide

Increasing Reactivity

RELATIVE STRENGTH OF COMMON ACIDS & THEIR CONJUGATE BASE

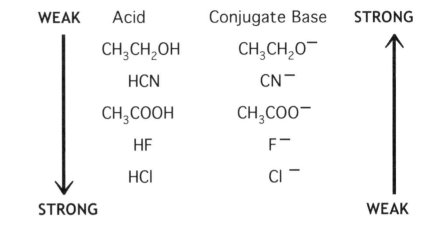

WEAK	Acid	Conjugate Base	STRONG
	CH_3CH_2OH	$CH_3CH_2O^-$	
	HCN	CN^-	
	CH_3COOH	CH_3COO^-	
	HF	F^-	
	HCl	Cl^-	
STRONG			WEAK

COMMON REACTIONS : Carboxylic Axids

AMIDES

```
     O                              O
     ||                             ||
     C                              C
R          OH  +  R₂NH   heat   R         NR₂  + H₂O
                          →
carboxylic acid   Amine                Amide
```

REACTIVITY OF LEAVING GROUP: S_N1 Reactions

$$H_2O > Cl^- > Br^- > I^- > TosO^-$$

Increasing Reactivity

SN₂ REACTIONS

Transition State

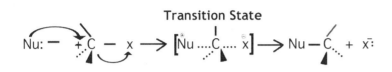

LEGEND:

Nu: = nucleophile

Y: = leaving group

STRUCTURE OF FRUCTOSE

$$CH_2OH$$
$$C = O$$
$$HO - C - H$$
$$H - C - OH$$
$$H - C - OH$$
$$CH_2OH$$

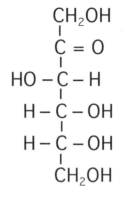

D - Fructose

D - Fructose
(Furanose Form)

SAPONIFACTION

... is the reaction through which fats
and glycerides are hydrolyzed

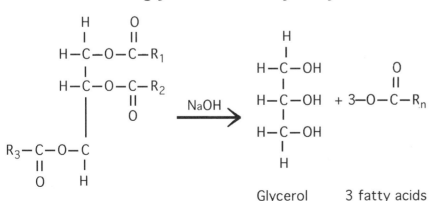

Triacyl Glyceride

Glycerol   3 fatty acids

S$_N$2 REACTIONS

Transition State

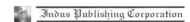

$$Nu:^- + \; C - Y \longrightarrow [\ominus Nu ... C ...Y \ominus]$$

LEGEND:

Nu:$^-$ = nucleophile

Y: = leaving group

$$Nu \quad C + Y:$$

SUBSTITUTED AROMATIC RINGS

ORTHO- AND PARA-DIRECTING DEACTIVATORS

- F
- Cl   } Halogens
- Br
- I

TETRAHEDRAL

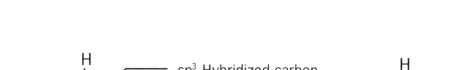

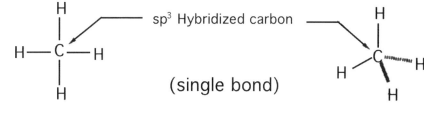

(single bond)

STRUCTURE OF GLUCOSE

D - Glucose

D - Glocose

(pyranose Form)

SUBSTITUTED AROMATIC RINGS

ORTHO - AND PARA-DIRECTING ACTIVATORS

- $\ddot{O}H$

- CH_3

- $\ddot{N}HCOCH_3$

GAS LAWS: Boyle's Law

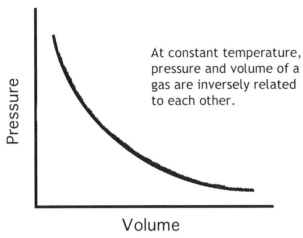

At constant temperature, pressure and volume of a gas are inversely related to each other.

Constant Temperature
PV = Constant

Centripetal Force and Acceleration

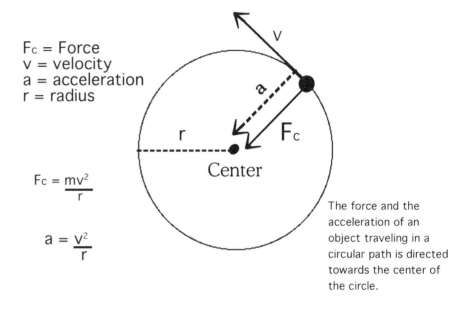

F_c = Force
v = velocity
a = acceleration
r = radius

$$F_c = \frac{mv^2}{r}$$

$$a = \frac{v^2}{r}$$

The force and the acceleration of an object traveling in a circular path is directed towards the center of the circle.

Atomic Structure

ORGANIZATION OF ELECTRONS IN ATOMS

Number of shell		Maximum number of electrons
FIRST SHELL	(1)	2
SECOND SHELL	(2)	8
THIRD SHELL	(3)	18
FOURTH SHELL	(4)	32

INCREASING ENERGY

Number of Electrons = $2n^2$

CENTER OF MASS

If two masses, m_1 amd m_2 lie at positions $x = x_1$, and $x = x_2$, respectively, then their center of mass is at position

$$x_{cm} = \bar{x} = \frac{m_1x_1 + m_2x_2}{m_1 + m_2}$$

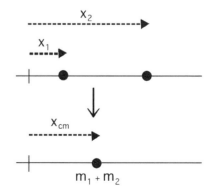

CONCAVE MIRROR

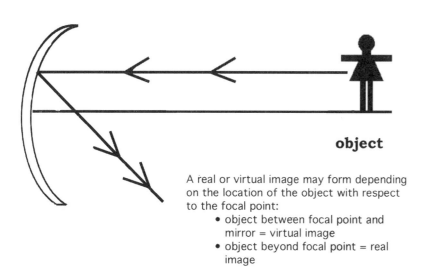

object

A real or virtual image may form depending on the location of the object with respect to the focal point:
- object between focal point and mirror = virtual image
- object beyond focal point = real image

CONCAVE MIRRORS & IMAGES

OBJECT POSITION	IMAGE TYPE	IMAGE SIZE	IMAGE
At F	No Image	–	–
At C	Real	Inverted	Same Size
Beyond C	Real	Inverted	Smaller
In Front of F	Virtual	Erect	Larger

CONCAVE LENS: Diverging

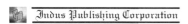

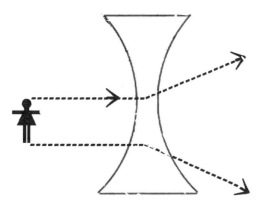

All images formed are virtual and direct.

CONCAVE MIRROR

FOCAL LENGTH • FOCAL POINT • CENTER OF CURVATURE

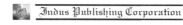

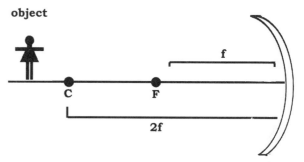

object

f

C   F

2f

f = focal Length

F = focal Point

C = center of Curvature

CONVEX LENS: Converging

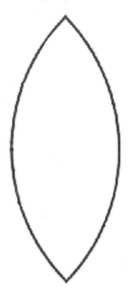

CONVERGING LENS

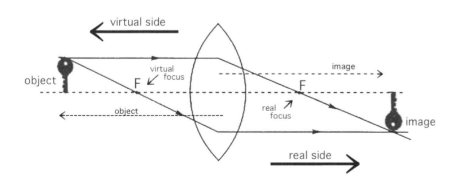

Image Type: Real & Inverted

CONVEX MIRROR

FOCAL LENGTH • FOCAL POINT • CENTER OF CURVATURE

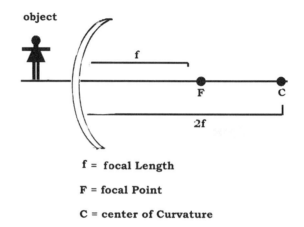

f = focal Length

F = focal Point

C = center of Curvature

CONVEX MIRROR

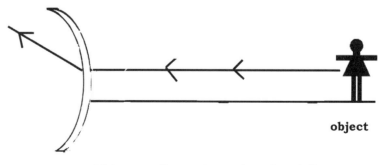

All images formed are virtual and direct

DISPLACEMENT

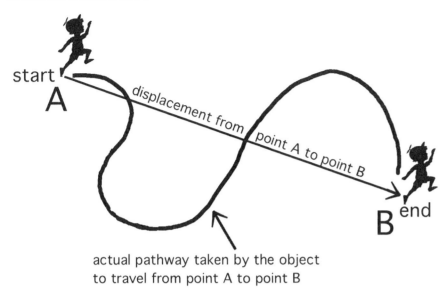

start

A

displacement from point A to point B

B end

actual pathway taken by the object
to travel from point A to point B

ELECTRIC CHARGE

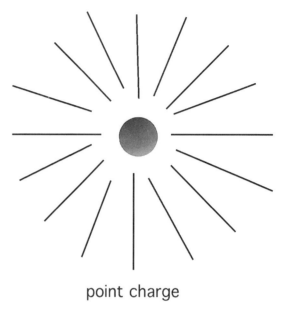

point charge

CONVEX MIRRORS & IMAGES

All images formed are virtual and erect.
The image is always formed behind the
mirror, and smaller in size with respect
to the size of the object.

EINSTEINS'S FAMOUS EQUATION

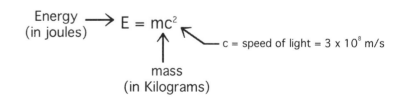

Energy
(in joules) → $E = mc^2$ ← c = speed of light = 3 x 10^8 m/s

mass
(in Kilograms)

ELECTRIC FIELD

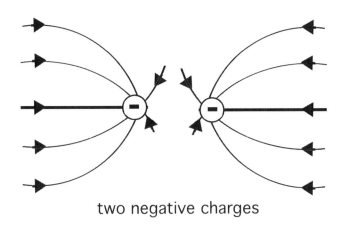

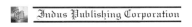

two negative charges

ELECTRIC FIELD: Around Charged Objects

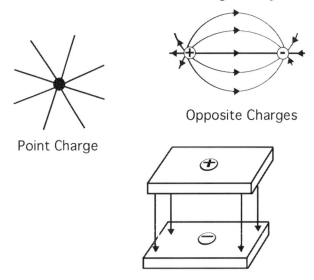

Point Charge

Opposite Charges

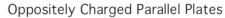

Oppositely Charged Parallel Plates

ELECTRIC FIELD

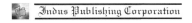

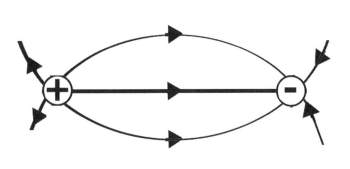

opposite charges

ELECTRIC FIELD

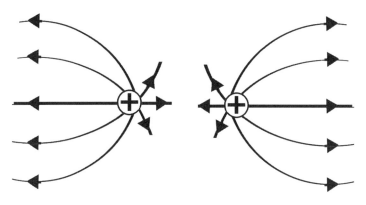

two positive charges

FORMULA SUMMARY: Electromagnetism

$P = IV$

$P = I^2R$

$P = \dfrac{V^2}{R}$

$W = Pt$

$W = VIt$

$W = I^2Rt$

P = power

I = current

V = electric potential

W = work (energy)

R = resistace

t = time

ENERGY AND CHARGED PLATES

OPPOSITELY CHARGED PLATES

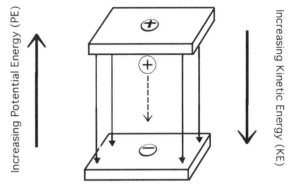

Oppositely Charged Parallel Plates

FORMULA SUMMARY: Electromagnetism

$F = \dfrac{kq_1q_2}{r^2}$

$E = F/q$

$V = W/q$

$E = V/d$

$R = V/I$

$I = \Delta q/\Delta t$

F = force

I = current

V = electric potential

W = work (energy)

q = charge

d = distance between charged plates

Series Circuits: $V_t = V_1 + V_2 + V_n$ $R_t = R_1 + R_2 + R_n$

   $I_t = I_1 = I_2 = I_n$

Parallel Circuits: $V_t = V_1 = V_2 = V_n$ $\dfrac{1}{R_t} = \dfrac{1}{R_1} + \dfrac{1}{R_2} + \dfrac{1}{R_n}$

   $I_t = I_1 + I_2 + I_n$

ENERGY: Pendulum

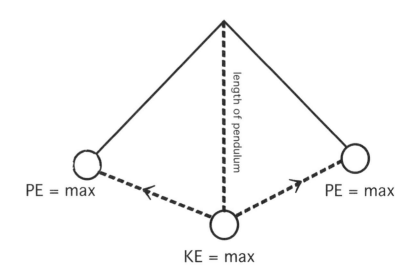

PHYSICS: Fluid Dynamics

BERNOULLI'S THEOREM

$$P_1 + \tfrac{1}{2}\rho v_2 + \rho gy = \text{Constant}$$

$$P_1 + \tfrac{1}{2}\rho v_2 + \rho gy = P_2 + \tfrac{1}{2}\rho v_2 + \rho gy$$

According to Bernoulli's theorem, given the height (y) is constant:
pressure and velocity are inversely related to each other.

MECHANICS: Force Inclined Plane

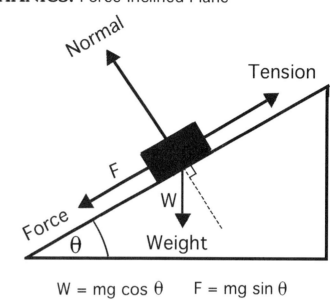

$$W = mg \cos \theta \qquad F = mg \sin \theta$$

ENERGY AND CHARGED PLATES

OPPOSITELY CHARGED PLATES

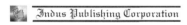

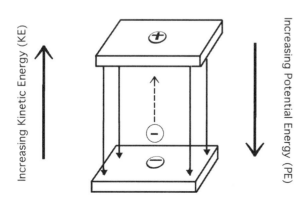

Oppositely Charged Parallel Plates

FLUIDS: Specific Gravity

SPECIFIC GRAVITY: is calculated as the weight of an object in air divided by the weight loss in water. specific gravity = weight in air / loss of weight

DENSITY: is expressed as mass divided by volume.
$$D\ (\rho) = M\ (\text{mass}) / V\ (\text{volume})$$

FORMULA SUMMARY: Internal Energy

$q = mc\Delta T$ q = amount of heat
             m = mass
             c = specific heat
$q = mHf$ T = temperature
                 (in Celsius degree)
$q = mHv$ Hf = heat of fusion
             Hv = heat of vaporization

SOUND: Interference & Resonance

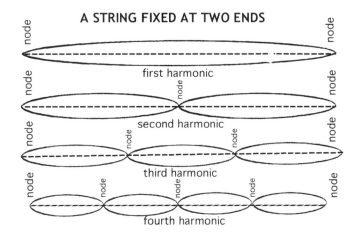

A STRING FIXED AT TWO ENDS

node — node (first harmonic)

node — node (second harmonic)

node — node (third harmonic)

node — node (fourth harmonic)

Node: the region where waves interfere to produce zero displacement.

Resonant wavelength: $\lambda_n = \dfrac{2L}{n}$ (n = 1,2,3 ...)

FORMULA SUMMARY: Electromagnetism

$F = qvB$ F = force
$V = \dfrac{F}{qv}$ B = magnetic flux
                 (or field strength)
$F = ilB$ V = electric potential
             l = length of the wire
             v = velocity
             i = current

FORMULA SUMMARY: Optics

$n = \dfrac{c}{v}$ c = speed of light in space (vacuum)
             f = frquency
$v = f\lambda$ n = index of refraction
$T = \dfrac{1}{f}$ l = wave length
             q = angle
$n_1 v_1 = n_2 v_2$ c = critical angle
$n_1 \sin\theta_1 = n_2 \sin\theta_2$ T = period
$\sin\theta_c = \dfrac{1}{n}$

Forces: Law Of Gravition

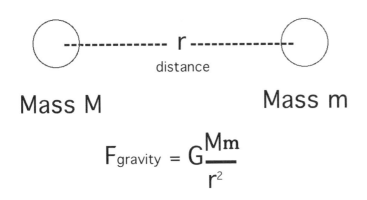

$$F_{gravity} = G\frac{Mm}{r^2}$$

The force is indirectly proportional to the square of the distance between two masses (negative slope on a graph).

THE PERIODIC TABLE: Ionization Energy Trend

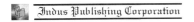
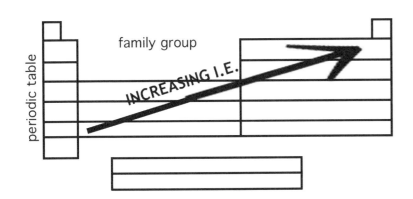

MECHANICS: Distance vs Time Graph

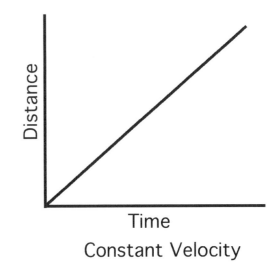

Constant Velocity

MECHANICS: Forced Plane

$$F = mg\ \sin\theta$$
(along the inclined plane)

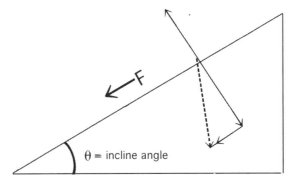

The trick to sloving inclined plane problems is to draw a similar triangle inside the larger triangle.

MECHANICS: Distance vs Time Graph

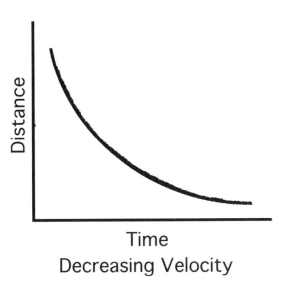

Decreasing Velocity

ELECTRICITY: Parallel Circuit

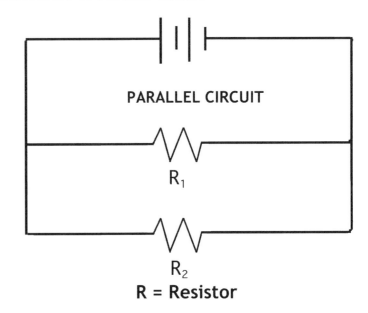

R = Resistor

MECHANICS: Distance vs Time Graph

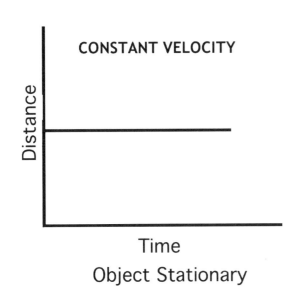

Object Stationary

ELECTRICAL: Series Circuit

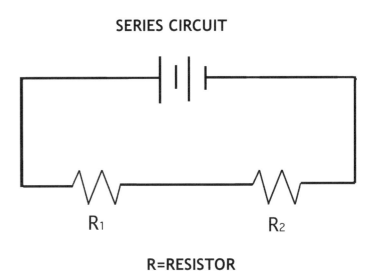

R=RESISTOR

PHYSICS: Projectile Motion

CHARACTERISTICS OF A PROJECTILE ALONG ITS PATHWAY:

MAXIMUM HEIGHT: is reached at 90°

MIMIMUM HEIGHT: is reached at 0°

MAXIMUM DISTANCE: when projectile is released at 45°

Total flight time: 2x flight time to reach the maximum height.

Max height = $v_0t + \frac{1}{2}gt^2$

PHYSICS: Wrap-Up

LIMITED REAGENTS

1. In order to determine the limiting reagent, a balanced equation is essential.
2. To figure out limiting reagents, you must understand stoichiometry.
3. Calculate the amount of moles or grams you would get for each reactant given. The one that gives you the smallest amount is the limiting reagent. The other(s) is in excess.
4. To calculate the amount of excess, calculate how many grams of the non-limiting reagent is needed to completely react with your limiting reagent. Subtract this from the amount you started with and the difference is the amount of excess left over.
5. The percent yield can be calculated by dividing the actual yield by the theoretical yield, then multipling by 100%.

PHYSICS: Momemtum

momentum = p = mv   (m=mass   v-velocity)

Total systemic energy is always conserved when two objects collide with each other.

$m_1v_1 + m_2v_2 = m_1v_1 + m_2v_2$ m_1 = mass $_1$ v_1=velocity
before collision   after collision m_2 = mass $_2$ v_2=velocity

COMPLETE INELASTIC COLLISION: objects stick without bouncing off each other following a collision.

COMPLETE ELASTIC COLLISION: objects bounce of each other following a collision.

CIRCUITS: Resistor

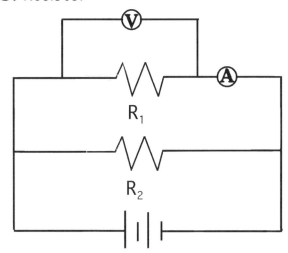

$\frac{1}{R} = \frac{1}{R_1} + \frac{1}{R_2}$ **Parallel Circuit**

PHYSICS: Plane Mirror

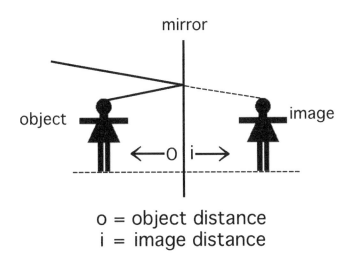

mirror

object   image

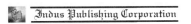

$\leftarrow$ o | i $\rightarrow$

o = object distance
i = image distance

REFLECTION

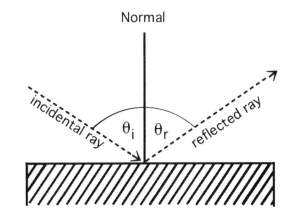

Normal

incidental ray θ_i | θ_r reflected ray

angle of incidence (θ_i) = angle of reflection (θ_r)

SUMMARY

STOICHIOMETRY

1. The key to Stoichiometry is a) have a good grasp of Dimensional Analysis and b) make sure your equation is balanced.
2. Stoichiometry is just a "reaction ratio," which is determined by the coefficents (those numbers that come before each compound in a balanced equation).
3. This reaction ratio is the only way you can go from one compound to another within any Dimensional Analysis calculation. And it is important to remember that this ratio is in MOLES, so you have to convert everything to moles first.

PROJECTILE MOTION

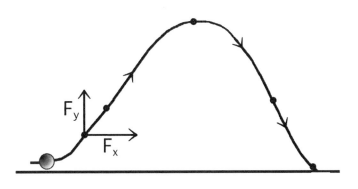

F_y

F_x

VERTICAL COMPONENT (F_y) = V• sin θ

HORIZONYAL COMPONENT (F_x) = V• cos θ

OPTICS: Refraction

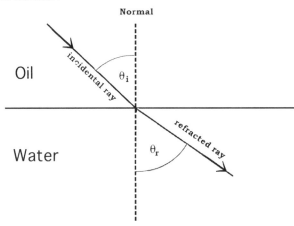

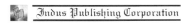

When light travels from a medium with a lower index
of refraction to a medium with a higher index of refraction:
the angle of incidence (θ_i) > the angle of refraction (θ_r)

OPTICS: Refraction

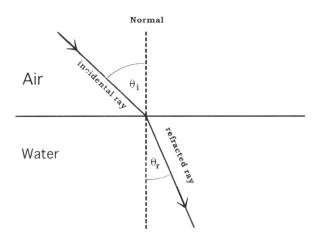

When light travels from a medium with a lower index
of refraction to a medium with a higher index of refraction:
the angle of incidence (θ_i) > the angle of refraction (θ_r)

PHYSICS: Resistor

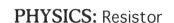
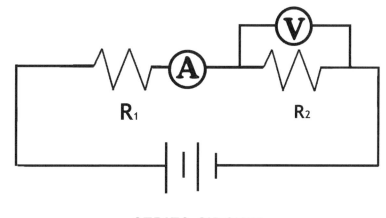

SERIES CIRCUIT

$$R_t = R_1 + R_2$$

RESOLVING COMPONENTS

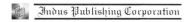
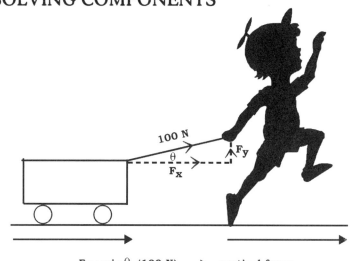

$F_y = \sin\theta$ (100 N) $\longrightarrow$ vertical force

$F_x = \cos\theta$ (100 N) $\longrightarrow$ hortizontal force

WAVES: Sine Wave

$$V = \lambda f$$

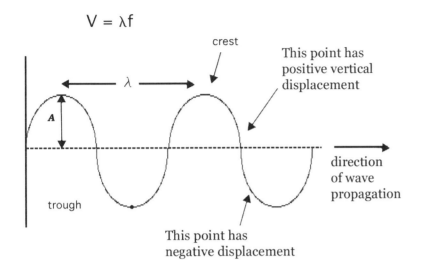

STANDING WAVES OF DIFFERENT WAVE LENGTHS: (along a string)

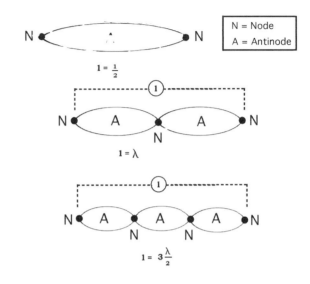

SIMPLE HARMONIC MOTION: Hooke's Law

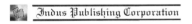

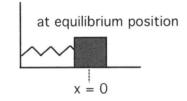

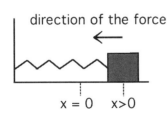 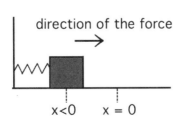

$$F = -kx$$

$$KE = \underline{1}\,kx^2$$

k = spring constant
x = displacement

SOUND: Longitudinal Waves

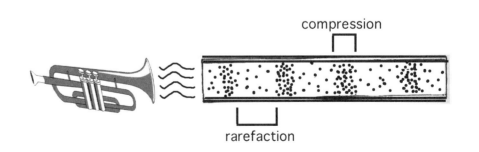

Sound waves (longitudinal) are created by alternating compression and expansion of air molecules.

FORMULA SUMMARY: Modern Physics

$E_{photon} = hf$
$W = hf_o$
$KE_{max} = hf - W$

$P = h/\lambda$
$E_{photon} = E_i - E_f$

E = energy
h = Planck's constant
f = frequency
f_o = threshold frequency
W = work
P = momentum
KE = kinetic energy

SUMMARY OF EQUATIONS: Energy

$\Delta PE = mg\Delta h$

$F = -kx$

$PE = \frac{1}{2} kx^2$

$KE = \frac{1}{2} mv^2$

F = force
PE = Potential Energy
KE = Kinetic Energy
k = Spring Constant
x = Change in the length of spring (displacement)
v = Velocity
m = Mass
g = Acceleration due to gravity

FORMULA SUMMARY: Energy

$PE = mgh$
$KE = \frac{1}{2}mv^2$
$KE = \frac{1}{2}kx^2$ (spring)
$W = Fd$
$P = Fv$
$P = W/\Delta t$
$P = Fd/t$

t = time
d = distance
v = velocity
h = height
P = power
F = force
ρ = momentum
W = work (energy)
PE = potential energy
KE = kinetic energy
x = displacement
g = 9.8 m/sec2
m = mass

SUMMARY OF EQUATIONS: Energy

$W = F\Delta d$

$P = \dfrac{W}{\Delta t} = \dfrac{F\Delta d}{\Delta t} = F\bar{v}$

W = work
F = force
Δt = time
d = distance

SUMMARY OF EQUATIONS: Series Circuits

$$V_t = V_1 + V_2 + V_3 + V_n$$

V = Voltage

$$I_t = I_1 = I_2 = I_3 = I_n$$

I = Current

$$\frac{1}{R_t} = \frac{1}{R_1} + \frac{1}{R_2} + \frac{1}{R_3} + \frac{1}{R_n}$$

R = Resistance

FORMULA SUMMARY: Mechanics

$$d = vt$$
$$v = d/t$$
$$a = \triangle v / \triangle t$$
$$d = v_i t + \tfrac{1}{2} a t^2$$
$$v_f^2 = v_i^2 + 2ad$$
$$V_f = v_i + at$$
$$F = ma$$
$$W = mg$$
$$I = F \triangle t$$
$$p = mv$$

d = distance
v = velocity
a = acceleration
v_i = velocity initial
v_f = velocity final
p = momentum
F = force
g = acceleration due to gravity
I = impulse
W = weight

SUMMARY OF EQUATIONS: Parallel Circuits

$$V_t = V_1 = V_2 = V_3 + V_n$$

V = Voltage

$$I_t = I_1 + I_2 + I_3 + I_n$$

I = Current

$$R_T = R_1 + R_2 + R_3 + R_n$$

R = Resistance

SUMMARY OF EQUATIONS: E & M

$$F = \frac{kq_1 q_2}{r^2}$$

$$E = \frac{F}{q}$$

$$E = \frac{v}{d}$$

F = Force
E = Electric Field
V = Charge
r = Distance
V = Voltage

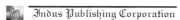

THE CIS / TRANS CONFIGURATION

CIS: substituents on the same side of the double bond.

TRANS: substituents on the opposite sides of the double bond.

H₃CH₂C ... CH₂CH₃
C = C
H ... H

Cis - 3 - pentene

H₃CH₂C ... H
C = C
H ... CH₂CH₃

Trans - 3 - Pentene

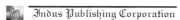

THE DIGESTIVE TRACT

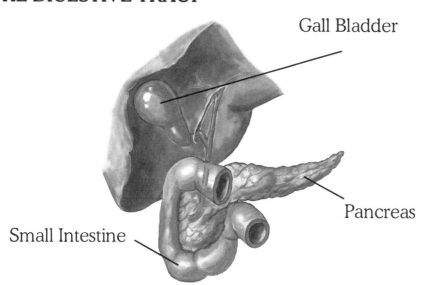

Gall Bladder

Pancreas

Small Intestine

 Indus Publishing Corporation

7052 Pokey Moonshine
Wayland, New York
14572

716-728-5752

MCAT: The Answer Key

 Indus Publishing Corporation

7052 Pokey Moonshine
Wayland, New York
14572

716-728-5752

Questions or Comments
write or e-mail:

induspub@aol.com

or visit our website:
www.induspublishing.com

GAS LAWS: Pressure vs. Temperature

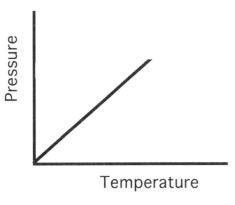

Volume Is Constant

At constant volume, the pressure and temperature of gas are directly related to each other.

DEFINITIONS

CONCAVE LENS: also known as diverging lens.

CONVEX LENS: also known as converging lens.

COULOMB'S LAW: is the electrostatic force between two points charges.
$$F = \frac{q_1 q_2}{r_2}$$

CRITICAL ANGLE: is the angle incident ray forms with the normal at which the refracted ray forms a right angle (90°) with the normal.

DISPERSION: is the phenomena in which light is separated into its spectrum.

TOTAL INTERNAL REFLECTION

$\theta_r = 90°$

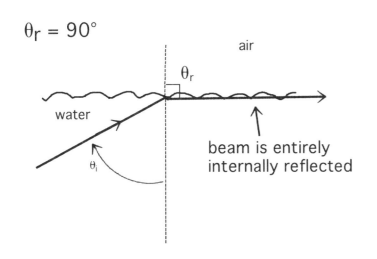

beam is entirely internally reflected

SUMMARY

PRECIPITATES

1. Precipitate and Acid-Base reactions are very similar. They are both double displacements, which means that they "swap" ions. In a precipitate reaction, you get a solid. In an acid-base reaction, you end up with water and a salt.

2. A combustion reaction involves some compound reacting with oxygen. You'll get three possible products, depending on what atoms are in you reactant.

3. A gas-forming reaction is a special type of double displacement, where either carbonic or sulfurous acid is formed, but breaks down further into carbon or sulfur dioxide, respectively. I should also note that simple swapping between an acid and a compound with sulfide, S_2, can also result in the immediate formation of a gas, $H_2S(g)$.

DEFINITIONS: Chemistry

MASS DEFECT: is the amount of matter transformed into energy when protons and neutrons combine to form a nucleus ($E=mc^2$)

MASS NUMBER: of an atom indicates the <u>sum</u> of protons and neutrons in its nucleus.

MIXTURE: is a substance formed by two or more compounds that are not chemically combined (ex: sand and pebbles is a mixture).

MOLALITY: is expressed as number of moles of solute per 1,000 grams of solvent (moles/g)

MOLAR VOLUME: is the volume occupied by <u>one mole</u> of a gas.

DEFINITIONS: CHEMISTRY

OXIDATION: is the process by which atoms <u>lose</u> an electron and in the process acquires a positive char<u>ge</u>.

OXIDIZING AGENT: causes other atoms to under go oxidation by accepting electrons. Oxidizing agents themselves are reduced during redox reactions.

PERIODS: are horizontal sequence of atoms in the Periodic Table.

POLAR MOLECULES: have partial charges due to asymmetrical charge distribution.

POTENTIAL ENERGY: also known as stored energy, is the measurement of an object's ability to do work.

DEFINITIONS: Chemistry

ABSOLUTE ZERO: the coldest temperature at which kinetic motion of molecules cease to exist (0°K or -273°C).

ACID: is a substance that can donate a proton (ex: Brönsted-Lowry acid).

ACTIVATION ENERGY: is the amount of energy required to start a reaction and form an activated complex.

ALKALI METALS: are metals that belong to Column 1 (IA) of the Periodic Table.

ALKALINE METALS: are metals that belong to Column 2 (IIA) of the Periodic Table.

DEFINITIONS: Chemistry

MOLE: consists of 6.02×10^{23} particles.

NEUTRALIZATION: is a reaction between an acid and a base that produce a salt and water as products.

NONELECTROLYTE: is an aqueous solution incapable of conducting electricity (no ions are present in an nonelectrolytic aqueous solution).

NONPOLAR COVALENT BOND: is a covalent bond in which two nonmetals share electrons equally between them.

OCTET: is the stable configuration of 8 valence electrons.

DEFINITIONS: Chemistry

SOLVENT: is the substance in which solutes are dissolved.

SPONTANEOUS REACTION: has low activation energy and continues to form products till one of the reactants is consumed.

STANDARD PRESSURE & TEMPERATURE (STP): 760 torr (1 atm) and 0°C.

STANDARD ELECTRODE POTENTIAL: The voltage of a half-cell in combination with a standard hydrogen cell.

STRONG ACIDS: have high acid ionization constant (K_a).

STRONG BASES: have high basic ionization constant (K_b).

DEFINITIONS: Chemistry

TRANSITIONAL ELEMENTS: have an incomplete d subshells.

VALENCE ELECTRONS: are the outermost electrons of an atom.

VAPOR PRESSURE: is the pressure exerted by the vapors of a liquid or a solid.

VOLT: is the unit measurement of electrical potential.

DEFINITIONS: Chemistry

PRECIPITATE: is the solid that is formed in a saturated solution when solutes are added to it.

REDOX: is the term used to describe a reduction-oxidation reaction.

REDUCTION: is the process by which atoms gain an electron and in the process acquires negative charge.

SOLUBILITY PRODUCT CONSTANT: $K_{sp} = [A_+][B-]$. The higher the K_{sp} the greater the solubility of the salt.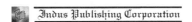

SOLUTE: are molecules that are dissolved in a solution.

DEFINITIONS: Chemistry

SUBLIMATION: is the process through which solids directly change into gases without going through the liquid phase (ex: dry ice).

SUPERSATURATED SOLUTIONS: have more solutes dissolved in them than saturated solution at the same temperature (note: by increasing the temperature, greater amounts of solutes can be dissolved in a given solvent).

TEMPERATURE: is the measure of the average kinetic energy of atoms that compose a substance (ex: gases).

TORR: is the unit measurement of pressure (standard pressure 760 torr=760 mm Hg).

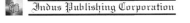
DEFINITIONS: Chemistry

BOND ENERGY: is the amount energy required to break a
chemical bond.

CALORIE: is the amount of heat needed to increase the
temperature of one gram of water by 1°C.

CATHODE: is the site of reduction in electrochemical cells.

CATION: is a positively charged ion.

CHARLES' LAW: states that volume and temperature of
gases are directly proportional to each other at
constant pressure.

DEFINITIONS: Chemistry

AVOGADRO'S HYPOTHESIS: states that all gases at the same
temperature and pressure contain the same number of
molecules.

AVOGADRO'S NUMBER: 6.02×10^{23} (the number of particles
in a mole).

AVOGADRO'S VOLUME: 22.4 L (the volume occupied by a mole
of gas at STP).

BASE: is a substance that can accept a proton (Brönsted-Lowery)
or donate hydroxide ion (OH-) in solution.

BOILING POINT ELEVATION: is the increase in the normal boiling point
of a substance due to addition of a solute.

DEFINITIONS: Chemistry

EXOTHERMIC REACTION: releases energy (heat) during reactions.
GROUPS: are vertically oriented chemically similar elements in
the Periodic Table.
FREEZING POINT DEPRESSION: is the decrease in the normal
freezing point of a substance due to addition of a solute.
HALOGENS: are set of elements grouped in Column 17 (VIIA)
of the Periodic Table.
HEAT OF FUSION: is the amount of heat absorbed by a substance
to change from the solid to the liquid phase without a
temperature change.
HETEROGENEOUS: is a mixture with uneven mix of substances.

DEFINITIONS: Chemistry

ELECTROLYTE: is a substance with dissolved ions in it. Conducts
electricity.

ELECTRONEGATIVITY: is the measurement of a nucleus' affinity
for electrons.

EMPIRICAL FORMULA: is the simplest representation of the elements
in a compound.

ENDOTHERMIC REACTION: absorbs energy (heat) during reactions.

END POINT: is the point during titration when neutralization is attained.

EQUILIBRIUM: is the point in a reversible reaction when both the
rates of forward and reverse reactions are the same.

NO BRAINER: Physics

WAVES III

- Single slit diffraction produces a much wider central maximum than double slit.
- As the frequency of a wave increases its energy increases and its wavelength decreases.
- Transverse wave particles vibrate back and forth perpendicular to the wave direction.
- Shorter waves with higher frequencies have shorter periods.
- Radiowaves are electromagnetic and travel at the speed of light (c).
- Monochromatic light has one frequency.
- Coherent light waves are all in phase.

DEFINITIONS: Chemistry

AMPHOTERIC SUBSTANCE: can act as both an acid (proton donor) and a base (proton acceptor).

ANION: is a negatively charged ion.

ANODE: is the site of oxidation in electrochemical cells.

AQUEOUS: is a term applied to all solutions with water as the solvent.

ATMOSPHERE (atm): is the unit measurement of pressure of gases.

ATOMIC NUMBER: is the number of protons in an atom.

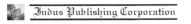

DEFINITIONS: Chemistry

HOMOGENOUS: is a substance with even mix of particles.

HYDROLYSIS: is a chemical reaction in which water is a reactant.

IDEAL GAS: is a gas that abides by all known gas laws (note: in reality there is no such thing as an ideal gas. Only H and He come close to acting as ideal gases.)

INERT GASES: also known as noble gases are found in column 18 of the Periodic Table.

IONIC BOND: is formed between a metal and a non-metal.

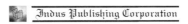

DEFINITIONS: Chemistry

IONIZATION ENERGY: is the amount of energy required to remove electron(s) from the valence shell of an electron.

ISOTOPES: are elements with different numbers of neutrons, but the same numbers of protons in their nuclei (mass numbers are different).

JOULE: is the unit measurement of energy (4.18 joules = 1 calorie)

KINETIC ENERGY: is the energy associated with motion (objects must be in motion to have a defined kinetic energy).

KINETIC THEORY: states that all gases under identical temperature and pressure behaves exactly alike.

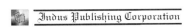
DEFINITIONS: Physics

Doppler Effect: is the apparent change in frequency and wave length when the source of sound/light and the observer move towards or away from each other.

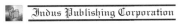
DEFINITIONS: PHYSICS

ANGLE OF REFRACTION: is the angle between a ray of light emerging from the interface of two media and the normal.

AVERAGE SPEED: is the total distance traveled by an object divided by the time traveled (scalar quantity).

BETA PARTICLE: is an electron that is spontaneously emitted from the nucleus of an atom.

BINDING ENERGY: is the amount of energy required to break up an nucleus into its individual components – protons and neutrons..

DEFINITIONS: Chemistry

COLLIGATIVE PROPERTIES: define a set of behaviors of solutions when solutes are added.

COMPOUND: is a substance that decomposes into two or more simpler molecules.

COVALENT BOND: is a bond formed between two non-metals.

DIPOLE: is a molecule with uneven charge distribution (partial charge).

DISTILLATION: is a process through which substances dissolved in solution are separated by boiling followed by recovery of vapors.

DEFINITIONS: Physics

BOYLE'S LAW: states that volume and pressure of a gas are inversely related to each other.

CENTER OF CURVATURE: is the point that is located at exactly the center of a spherical mirror.

CENTRIPETAL FORCE: is the minimum force required to keep an object moving in a circular path.

COEFFICIENT OF FRICTION: is the ratio between the force needed to overcome friction and the normal force joining two surfaces together.

MATHEMATICS: Algebra

RULES OF EXPONENTIAL ALGEBRA

$$X^a \bullet X^b = X^{a+b} \qquad X^a/X^b = X^{a-b} \qquad (X^a)^b = X^{ab}$$

$$X_0 = 1 \ (X \text{ is any real positive number}) \qquad X_{-1} = 1/X$$

$$X1/a = a \ X \qquad Xa/b = a \ X^b \qquad X-a/b = 1/a \ X^b$$

$$(X \bullet Y)^a = X^a \bullet Y^a \qquad (X/Y)^a = X^a/Y^a$$

MATHEMATICS: Definitions

AVERAGE: is the sum of two or more numbers divided by the number of those quantities. Ex: $n_1+n_2+n_3/3$ = average

AXIS: is an imaginary straight line around which an object is thought to rotate.

CONSTANT: is a symbol or number that represents the same value under all situations/conditions.

CRITICAL POINT: is a point on a graph that represents the derivative of a function that is equal to zero or infinity.

DEGREE: is the unit measurement for angles and arcs.

DEFINITIONS: Physics

ABSOLUTE ZERO: the theoretical lowest possible temperature on the Kelvin Scale.

ACCELERATION: is the vector quantity – the change of velocity divided by the change of time.

ALPHA DECAY: is the spontaneous expulsion of a helium ion from an atomic nucleus.

AMPERE: is the unit measurement of current.

ANGLE OF INCIDENCE: is the angle between a ray of light and the normal(normal is perpendicular to the surface where the light strikes).

MATHEMATICS: Definitions

EQUATION: represents a mathematical relationship between two or more variables.

MANTISSA: is the decimal portion of a logarithm.

MEDIAN: is the middle number in a series arranged in an ascending order. Ex: 3 4 5 7 9 (5 is the median).

MODE: is the value/number represented most frequently in a series of numbers. Ex: 3, 5, 13, 3, 9, 21, 3, 5 (3 is the mode).

RATIO: is a quotient formed as a result of one number divided by another.

SCALAR QUANTITY: is a real number, but has no defined direction. Ex: temperature

MNEMONICS: Chemistry

FAT-SOLUABLE VITAMINS

"ADEK"

Vitamins **A** ,**D**, **E**, and **K**

MNEMONICS: Chemistry

CITRIC ACID CYCLE

Oh   (Oxaloacetate)
Citric   (Citrate)
Acid   (Aconitate)
Is   (Isocitrate)
Of course   (Oxalosuccinate)
A   (alpha-ketoglutarate)
Silly   (Succinyl-CoA)
Stupid   (Succinate)
Funny   (Fumarate)
Molecule   (Malate)

MNEMONICS: Biology

MITOSIS

"**P**eople **M**eet **A**nd **T**alk"
Interphase + "PMAT"

Interphase, Prophase, Metaphase, Anaphase, Telophase.

(Note: 2 daughter cells are formed at the end of Mitosis.)

MNEMONICS: Chemistry

"**EX**ons **EX**pressed, **IN**trons **IN** the trash"
DNA expression into mature mRNA
Pyrimidines are "CUT" from purines.
Pyrimidines are Cytosine, Uracil, Thiamine
    and are one ring structures. Purines are
    double ring structures.

MNEMONICS: HUMAN PHYSIOLOGY

AUTONOMIC NERVOUS SYSTEM

SYMPATHETIC: fight or flight
(the only neurotransmitter used by the
sympathetic nervous system is norepinephrine.)

PARASYMPATHETIC: rest and digest
(there are two neurotransmitters involved with
the parasympathetic nervous system: acetylcholine
and norephinephrine.)

MNEMONICS: Human Physiology

CRANIAL NERVES

I	On (Olfactory)
II	Old (Optic)
III	Olympus (Oculomotor)
IV	Towering (Trochlear)
V	Tops, (Trigeminal)
VI	A (Abducens)
VII	Finn (Facial)
VIII	And (Auditory)
IX	German (Glossopharyngeal)
X	Viewed (Vagus)
XI	Astounding (Accessory)
XII	Hops (Hypoglossal)

MNEMONICS: Human Physiology

Hormones produced by the Anterior Pituitary Gland

"FLAGTOP"

F: Follicle Stimulating Hormone
L: Lutinizing Hormone
A: ACTH
G: Growth Hormone
T: Thyroid Stimulating Hormone
O: MSH
P: Prolactin

MNEMONICS: Human Physiology

OXYHEMOGLOBIN DISSOCIATION CURVE

Think of an exercising muscle for a rightward shift:
Exercising muscle is:
hot,
acidic (lactic acid),
hypercarbic,
and has increased 2,3-DPG.
It benefits from oxygen unloading from red blood cells.
Also think Bohr effect with a rightward shift($CO_2 = O_2$).
    Realize that the Haldane effect means
    ($O_2 = CO_2$ carried by Hgb).

MNEMONICS: Human Physiology

SPINAL NERVES

C3-4-5 keep the phrenic nerve (or diaphragm) alive

C5-6-7 raise your arms to heaven
(nerve roots of long thoracic nerve innervate
serratus anterior)

MNEMONICS: Human Physiology

BRANCHES OF THE FACIAL NERVE

"Ten Zombies Bought My Car"

Temporal, Zygomatic, Buccal, Masseteric, Cervical

MNEMONICS: Human Physiology

GREAT VESSELS OF THE HEART

ABC'S

Aortic arch gives rise to:
Brachiocephalic trunk,
the left Common Carotid
the left Subclavian artery

MNEMONICS: Human Physiology

CRANIAL BONES

"Old People From Texas Eat Spiders"

Occipital, Parietal, Frontal, Temporal, Ethnoid,
and Sphenoid

MNEMONICS: Biology

GLYCOLSIS

Goodness (Glucose)
Gracious, (Glucose-6-P)
Father (Fructose-6-P)
Franklin (Fructose-1, 6-diP)
Did (Dihydroxyacetone-P)
Go (Glyceraldehyde-P)
By (1,3-Biphosphoglycerate)
Picking (3-phosphoglycerate)
Pumpkins (2-phosphoglycerate)
to
Prepare (Phosphoenolpyruvate)
Pies (Pyruvate)

MATHEMATICS: Symbols

G	giga	10^9
M	mega	10^6
K	kilo	10^3
c	centi	10^{-2}
m	milli	10^{-3}
m	micro	10^{-6}
n	nano	10^{-9}
p	pico	10^{-12}

MNEMONICS: Biology

MEIOSIS

"PMAT x2"
1st cell division: Interphase, Prophase I, Metaphase I, Anaphase I, Telophase I
2nd cell division: Prophase II, Metaphase II, Anaphase II, Telophase II

(Note: 4 haploid daughter cells instead of 2 diploid daughter cells are produced at the end of meiosis.)

Important: There is no Interphase II.

MNEMONICS: Biology

CELL CYCLE

"Go Sally Go! Make Children!"
G_1, S, G_2, M, C

G_1 = Growth phase 1
S = DNA Synthesis (replication)
G_2 = Growth phase 2
M = Mitosis
C = Cytokinesis

MNEMONICS: Physics

BASIC PHYSICAL STANDARD MEASUREMENTS

"Taking Luxurious Limos More Noxious Than Cycling"

Temperature (K) = Kelvin
Length (m) = meter
Luminous intensity (Cd) = candles
Mass (kg) = kilogram
Number of particles (moles)
Time (s) = seconds
Charge (C) = Coulombs

NO BRAINER: Physics

ELECTRICITY

- Insulators contain no free electrons.
- Ionized gases conduct electric current using positive ions, negative ions and electrons.
- Electric fields all point in the direction of the force on a positive test charge.
- Electric fields between two parallel plates are uniform in strength except at the edges.
- Millikan determined the charge on a single electron using his famous oil-drop experiment.
- All charge changes result from the <u>movement</u> of electrons not protons. (ex: an object becomes positive by losing electrons)

MNEMONICS: Physics

REMEMBER FEW V

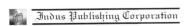

$$F = \frac{q\ q}{r}$$ drop an "r" → $$W = \frac{q\ q}{r}$$

drop a "q" ↓   drop a "q" ↓

$$E = \frac{q}{r}$$ drop an "r" → $$V = \frac{q}{r}$$

MNEMONICS: Physics

VISIBLE SPECTRUM

"**R**oy **G**. **B**iv" or
"**R**ichard **O**f **Y**ork **G**ained **B**attles **I**n **V**ain"

Red **O**range **Y**ellow **G**reen **B**lue **I**ndigo **V**iolet

* Red has the longest wavelength and the lowest frequency in the visible spectrum.

* Violet has the shortest wavelength and the highest frequency in the visible spectrum.

NO BRAINER: Physics

ENERGY

- Mechanical energy is the sum of the potential and kinetic energy.
- UNITS: $a=[m/sec^2]$, $F=[kg \bullet m/sec^2]$ (newton),
  work = pe = ke = $[kg \bullet m^2/sec^2]$ (joule)
- 1ev is an energy unit equal to $1.6 \times 10-19$ joules
- Gravitational potential energy increases as height increases.
- Kinetic energy changes only if velocity changes.
- Mechanical energy (pe + ke) does not change for a free falling mass or a swinging pendulum. *(air friction ignored)*
- Units for Power is [joules/sec] or the rate of change of energy.

NO BRAINER: Physics

MAGNETISM

- The direction of a magnetic field is defined by the direction a compass needle points.
- Magnetic fields point from the north to the south outside the magnet and south to north inside the magnet.
- Magnetic flux is measured in **webers.**
- Left hands are for negative charges and Right hands are for positive charges.
- The first hand rule deals with the B-field around a current bearing wire, the third hand rule looks at the force on charges moving in a B-field, and the second hand rule is redundant.
- Solenoids are stronger with more current or more wire turns or adding a soft iron core.

NO BRAINER: Physics

ELECTRICITY

- A coulomb is charge, an amp is current [coulomb/sec] and a volt is potential difference [joule/coulomb].
- Short, fat and cold wires make the best conductors.
- Electrons and protons have equal amounts of charge ($1.6 \times 10-19$ coulombs each).
- Adding a resistor in parallel *decreases* the total resistance of a circuit.
- Adding a resistor in series *increases* the total resistance of a circuit.
- All resistors *in series* have equal current **(I).**
- All resistors *in parallel* have equal voltage **(V).**
- If two charged spheres touch each other add the charges and divide by two to find the final charge on each sphere.

NO BRAINER: Physics

INTERNAL ENERGY

- Internal energy is the sum of temperature (ke) and phase (pe) conditions.
- Steam and liquid water molecules at 100 degrees have equal kinetic energies.
- Degrees Kelvin (absolute temp.) Is equal to zero degrees (0°) Celsius.
- Temperature measures the average kinetic energy of the molecules.
- Phase changes are due to potential energy changes.
- Internal energy always flows from an object at higher temperature to one of lower temperature.

NO BRAINER: Physics

MECHANICS

- Weight (force of gravity) decreases as you move away from the earth by distance squared.
- Mass and inertia are the same thing.
- Constant velocity and zero velocity means the net force is zero and acceleration is zero.
- Weight (in newtons) is mass x acceleration (w = mg).
  Mass is not Weight!
- Velocity, displacement [s], momentum, force and acceleration are vectors.
- Speed, distance [d], time, and energy (joules) are scalar quantities.

- The slope of the velocity-time graph is acceleration.

NO BRAINER: Physics

NUCLEAR PHYSICS

- Isotopes have different neutron numbers and atomic masses but the same number of protons (atomic numbers).
- Geiger counters, photographic plates, cloud and bubble chambers are all used to detect or observe radiation.
- Fusion requires that hydrogen be combined to make helium.
- Fission requires that a neutron causes uranium to be split into middle size atoms and produce extra neutrons.
- Radioactive half-lives <u>can not</u> be changed by heat or pressure.
- One AMU of mass is equal to 931 meV of energy. ($E = mc^2$).
- Nuclear forces are strong and short ranged.

NO BRAINER: Physics

MECHANICS

- At zero degrees (0°) two vectors have a resultant equal to their sum.
  At 180° two vectors have a resultant equal to their difference.
  From the difference to the sum is the total range of possible resultants.
- Centripetal force and centripetal acceleration vectors are toward the center of the circle- while the velocity vector is <u>tangent</u> to the circle.
- An unbalanced force (object not in equilibrium) must produce acceleration.
- The slope of the distance-tine graph is velocity.
- The <u>equilibrant</u> force is equal in magnitude but opposite in direction to the <u>resultant</u> vector.
- Momentum is conserved in all collision systems.
- Magnitude is a term use to state how large a vector quantity is.

PHYSICS: No Brainers

MODERN PHYSICS

- A photon is a particle of light *(wave packet)*.
- All electromagnetic waves originate from accelerating charged particles.
- The frequency of a light wave determines its energy (E = hf).
- The lowest energy state of a atom is called the ground state.
- Increasing light frequency increases the <u>kinetic</u> energy of the emitted photo-electrons.
- As the threshold frequency increase for a photo-cell (photo emissive material) the work function also increases.
- Increasing light intensity <u>increases</u> the number of emitted photo-electrons but not their KE.

NO BRAINER: PHYSICS

OPTICS

- Real images are always inverted.
- Virtual images are always upright.
- Diverging lens (concave) produce only small virtual images.
- Light rays bend away from the normal as they gain speed and a longer wavelength by entering a slower (n) medium {frequency remains constant}.
- The focal length of a converging lens (convex) is shorter with a higher (n) value lens or if blue light replaces red.

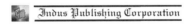

NO BRAINER: Physics

WAVES II

- Light wave are transverse (they can be polarized).
- The speed of all types of electromagnetic waves is 3.0 x 108 m/sec in a vacuum.
- The amplitude of a sound wave determines its energy.
- Constructive interference occurs when two waves are zero (0) degrees out of phase or a whole number of wavelengths (360 degrees.) out of phase.
- At the critical angle a wave will be refracted to 90 degrees.
- According to the Doppler effect a wave source moving toward you will generate waves with a shorter wavelength and higher frequency.
- Double slit diffraction works because of diffraction and interference.

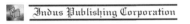

NO BRAINER: Physics

NUCLEAR PHYSICS

- Alpha particles are the same as helium nuclei and have the symbol.
- The atomic number is equal to the number of protons (2 for alpha)
- The number of nucleons is equal to protons + neutrons (4 for alpha)
- Only charged particles can be accelerated in a particle accelerator such as a cyclotron or Van Der Graaf generator.
- Natural radiation is alpha (a).beta (b) and gamma (high energy x-rays)
- A loss of a beta particle results in an increase in atomic number.
- All nuclei weigh less than their parts. This mass defect is converted into binding energy. ($E=mc^2$)

NO BRAINER: Physics

WAVES I

- Sound waves are longitudinal and mechanical.
- Light slows down, bends toward the normal and has a shorter wavelength when it enters a higher (n) value medium.
- All angles in wave theory problems are measured to the normal.
- Blue light has more energy. A shorter wavelength and a higher frequency than red light (remember – ROYGBIV).
- The electromagnetic spectrum (radio, infrared, visible. Ultraviolet x-ray and gamma) are listed lowest energy to highest.
- A prism produces a rainbow from white light by dispersion. (red bends the least because it slows the least).

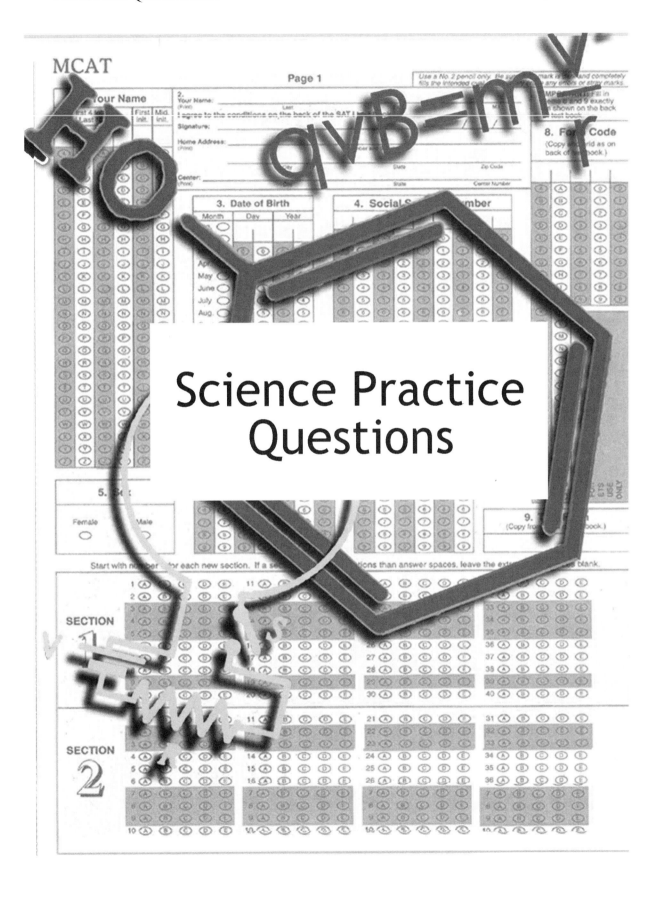

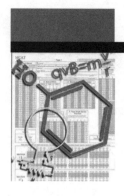

SCIENCE
PRACTICE QUESTIONS

THESE QUESTIONS ARE NOT IN MCAT FORMAT. THEY ARE INTENDED ONLY TO
TEST YOUR KNOWLEDGE OF THE SCIENCES

1) Of the quantities noted, which one is *not* a vector
quantity?
(A) velocity   (D) displacement
(B) torque   (E) kinetic energy
(C) momentum

2) A body on earth has mass, weight and rotational inertia.
Which of these properties change(s) when the body is
taken to another planet?
(A) only mass   (D) both rotational inertia and weight
(B) only weigh   (E) rotational inertia, mass and weight
(C) only rotational inertia

3) Which unit applies to the product of $\underline{1kg}$ x $\underline{1m}$ x $\underline{1}$ x $\underline{1m}$

$\qquad\qquad\qquad\qquad\qquad\qquad\quad$ 1 $\qquad$ 1s $\quad$ 1s $\quad$ 1

(A) Newton   (C) slug   (E) $kg{\cdot}m / s^2$
(B) Joule   (D) watt

4) How many square centimeters are there in exactly one square
meter?
(A) 10^2 (C) 10^4 (E) none of these
(B) 10^{-2} (D) 10^{-4}

5) Which set of displacement vectors *could not* be combined to yield a resultant of magnitude 68cm?
   (A) 22 cm and 46 cm   (C) 44 cm and 49 cm   (E) 74 cm and 28 cm
   (B) 88 m and 32 cm   (D) 93 cm and 10 cm

6) Which expression is *not true* concerning the vectors shown in the sketch to the right?
   (A) C = A + B   (D) C < A + B
   (B) C + A = -B   (E) A² + B² = C²
   (C) A + B + C = 0

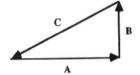

Questions 7 through 10 pertains to the statement below:

Starting from rest, a particle which is confined to move along a straight line is accelerated at a rate of 4.0 m/s²

7) Which statement accurately describes the motion of this particle?
   (A) The particle travels 4.0 m during each second.
   (B) The particle travels 4.0 m *only* during the first second.
   (C) The speed of the particle increases by 4.0 m/s² during each second.
   (D) The acceleration of the particle increases by 4.0 m/s² during each second.
   (E) The final velocity of the particle will be proportional to the distance that the particle covers.

8) After 10 seconds, how far will the particle have traveled?
   (A) 20 m   (C) 100 m   (E) 400 m
   (B) 40 m   (D) 200 m

9) What is the speed of the particle after it has traveled 8.0 m?
   (A) 4.0 m/s   (C) 8 m/s   (E) 100 m/s
   (B) 40 m   (D) 200 m

10) Which statement concerning the *slope of the position versus time graph* for this particle is true?
(A) It is both negative and constant.
(B) It has a constant value of 4.0 m/s.
(C) It has a constant value of 4.0 m/s^2.
(D) It is *not* constant and *increases* with increasing time.
(E) It is *not* constant and *decreases* with increasing time.

Questions 11 through 15 pertain to the situation described below.

The drawing below shows the timer marks on a tape that was pulled by a cart which moved on an air track. The timer marks were made at equal time intervals of 0.05 s. Five of the timer marks are labeled A through E for identification purposes. A centimeter scale is shown below the tape for measurement purposes.

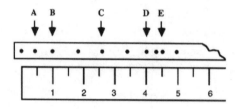

11) At which of the marked points was the velocity of the cart the greatest?
(A) A   (C) C   (E) E
(B) B   (D) D

12) At which of the marked points was the net force on the object most likely to be equal to zero?
(A) A   (C) C   (E) E
(B) B   (D) D

13) What was the average velocity of the object over the first 4.0 cm?
(A) 1.3cm/s   (C) 10.0 cm/s   (E) 13.3 cm/s
(B) 8.9cm/s   (D) 11.4 cm/s

14) Determine the displacement of the object *during the third time interval.*
(A) 0.05 cm   (C) 10.0cm/s   (E) 1.8 cm
(B) 0.20 cm   (D) 1.0 cm

15) Which is the best estimate of the instantaneous velocity of the object at 0.20 s ?
(A) 1.6cm/s   (C) 9.0 cm/s   (E) 16 cm/s
(B) 2.6cm/s   (D) 13 cm/s

16) The graph below shows the velocities of two bodies A and B, as functions of time.

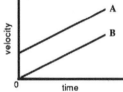

When mass **A** is acted upon by a force. it is accelerated at a rate of 3.0m/s². When mass **B** is acted upon by a the same force, it is accelerated at at rate of 1.5m/s². What is the relationship between the ,masses?
(A) $2m_A = m_B$ (C) $4m_A = m_B$ (E) $m_A = m_B$
(B) $m_A = 2m_B$ (D) $m_A = 4m_B$

17) Which physical quantity *must* be the same for both bodies?
(A) mass   (C) inertia   (E) applied force
(B) weight   (D) acceleration

Questions 18 through 21 pertain to the statement below:

A 2.0 kg projectile is fired at an angle of 60° with respect to the horizontal with an initial speed of 30 m/s.

18) Which entry in the table below correctly describes the initial velocity of the projectile?

	Horizontal Component	Vertical Component
(A)	15 m/s	26 m/s
(B)	30 m/s	52 m/s
(C)	26 m/s	15 m/s
(D)	52 m/s	30 m/s
(E)	30 m/s	30 m/s

19) How far will the projectile travel *horizontally* at the end of 2.0s?
    (A) 15 m   (C) 36 m   (E) 60 m
    (B) 30 m   (D) 53 m

20) How long does it take the projectile to reach the highest point in its path?
    (A) 1.5 s   (C) 3.1 s   (E) 9.8 s
    (B) 2.7 s   (D) 6.2 s

21) Determine the kinetic energy of the projectile when it reaches the highest point in its trajectory.
    (A) zero   (C) 676 J   (E) none of these
    (B) 225 J   (D) 900 J

22) Which is characteristic of an *inelastic* collision?
    (A) total mass is not conserved
    (B) total energy is not conserved
    (C) kinetic energy is not conserved
    (D) linear momentum is not conserved
    (E) the total impulse is equal to the change in the kinetic energy

Questions 23 and 24 pertain to the statement on the next page:

A horse pulls a cart along a flat level road. Consider the following four forces which arise in this situation:

F_A = the force of the horse pulling on the cart

F_B = the force of the cart pulling on the horse

F_C = the force of the horse pulling on the road

F_D the force of the road pulling on the horse

23) Which two forces form an "action-reaction" pair which obeys Newton's third law?
(A) F_A and F_D (C) 5 lb   (E) none of these
(B) F_B and F_C (D) F_C and F_D

24) Suppose that the horse and cart have started from rest and as time goes on, their speed increases. Which can be concluded concerning the magnitudes of the forces mentioned above?
(A) $F_A > F_B$ (C) $F_B > F_D$ (E) $F_A + F_D$
(B) $F_B < F_C$ (D) $F_C > F_D$

25) A 3 lb block is placed on top of a 5 lb block that is in a stable position on a table. What is the magnitude of the force exerted by the table on the 5 lb block?
(A) 2 lb   (C) 5 lb   (E) none of these
(B) 3 lb   (D) 8 lb

26) What force is required to lift a 10 kg block *vertically upward* with an acceleration of 2 m/s²?
(A) 20 N   (C) 98 N   (E) 118 N
(B) 78 N   (D) 100 N

27) A rock is suspended from a rope and moves downward at constant speed. Which statement is true concerning the tension in the rope?
(A) It is zero.
(B) It points downward.
(C) It has the same magnitude as the weight of the rock.
(D) Its magnitude is less than that of the weight of the rock.
(E) Its magnitude is greater than that of the weight of the rock.

28) Which force is responsible for holding a car in an *unbanked* curve?
(A) The car's weight.
(B) The force of friction.
(C) The reaction force to the car's weight.
(D) The vertical component of the normal force.
(E) The horizontal component of the normal force.

Questions 29 and 30 pertain to the statement below:

A 2.0 N force acts horizontally on a 10 N block which is initially at rest on a horizontal surface. The coefficient of static friction between the block and the surface is 0.50.

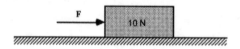

29) What is the magnitude of the frictional force which acts on the block?
(A) zero   (C) 5.0 N   (E) none of these
(B) 2.0 N   (D) 8.0 N

30) Suppose that the block now moves across the surface with constant speed under the action of a horizontal 3.0 N force. Which statement concerning this situation is *not* true?
(A) The net force on the block is zero.
(B) The acceleration of the block is zero.
(C) The frictional force on the block has magnitude 3.0 N.
(D) The coefficient of kinetic friction between the block and the surface is 0.30.
(E) The direction of the force that the surface exerts on the block is vertically upward.

31) A 2.0 N rock slides on a *frictionless* inclined plane.

Which statement is true concerning the *net force* that acts on the rock?
(A) It is zero.
(B) It is 2.0 N
(C) It is greater than 2.0N
(D) It is less than 2.0 N but greater than zero
(E) It *decreases* as the angle of incline is *increased*.

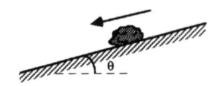

32) Consider the following four forces:
   (1) the force of gravity exerted on a falling stone
   (2) the force of air resistance exerted on a falling stone
   (3) the elastic force exerted on a block by a spring
   (4) the force of friction between two rough surfaces

Which of these is (are) conservative?
(A) 1 only   (C) both 1 and 3   (E) 1,2, and 3
(B) 3 only   (D) both 1 and 4

33) What does the area under a graph of *net force versus time* represent?
(A) velocity   (D) change in kinetic energy
(B) work done   (E) change in linear momentum
(C) displacement

34) A rocket orbits earth at constant speed in a circular path as shown in the figure below.

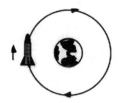

Note the arrows shown below:

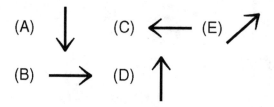

At the instant shown in the figure, which arrow represents the direction of the acceleration of the rocket?

   (A) A   (C) C   (E) E
   (B) B   (D) D

35) A car which initially possesses 4×10^5J of kinetic energy is brought to stop in 10 seconds over a distance of 40 m. How much work was done in stopping the car?

(A) zero   (D) 4×10^6J
(B) 4×10^4J   (E) cannot be determined from the information given
(C) 4×10^5J

36) Of the systems noted, which is nearly at its maximum potential energy?

(A) a run down clock
(B) water at the top of a dam
(C) a rock at the bottom of a cliff
(D) an unstretched spring
(E) a bowling ball rolling down an alley

Questions 37 and 38 pertain to the situation described below?

A 1500 kg car travels at a constant speed of 22 m/s around a circular track which is 80 meters in diameter.

37) Determine the magnitude of the centripetal force which acts on the car.
(A) 6.1 N
(B) 12.2 N
(C) 9.1×10^3 N
(D) 1.8×10^4 N
(E) none of these

38) What is the kinetic energy of the car?
(A) 1.6×10^4 J
(B) 3.3×10^4 J
(C) 3.6×10^5 J
(D) 7.2×10^5 J
(E) none of these

39) Which statement best explains why the centripetal force does not change the speed of the car?
(A) The centripetal force is a *pseudo* force.
(B) The centripetal force is equal to mv^2/r.
(C) The centripetal force produces no acceleration.
(D) The centripetal force is canceled by its "reaction" force.
(E) The centripetal force is always perpendicular to the velocity of the car.

40) How much time is required for a net force of 10 N to change the speed of a 5 kg mass by 3 m/s?
(A) 1.5 s
(B) 6.0 s
(C) 16.7 s
(D) 150.0 s
(E) 200 s

Questions 41 and 42 pertain to the situation below:

A space vehicle of mass M has speed v. At some instant, it separates into two pieces, each of mass M/2. One of the pieces is at rest just after the separation.

41) Which statement is true concerning this situation?
    (A) The moving piece has speed 2v.
    (B) This process conserves kinetic energy.
    (C) The piece at rest possesses kinetic energy.
    (D) This process does not conserve total energy.
    (E) This process does not conserve linear momentum.

42) Determine the kinetic energy of the moving piece just after
    separation.
    (A) zero   (C) $\frac{1}{2} Mv^2$ (E) $2 Mv^2$

    (B) $\frac{1}{4} Mv^2$ (D) Mv^2

43) The law of conservation of linear momentum applies to a
    two-body collision *only if*
    (A) all the collisions are elastic.
    (B) the net external impulse is zero.
    (C) the kinetic energy of the system is conserved.
    (D) the sum of the external torque's acting on the system is
        zero.
    (E) there is no increase or decrease in the internal energy of
        the system.

44) A non-zero torque is required to
    (A) produce a linear acceleration.
    (B) maintain a constant angular velocity.
    (C) produce a change in angular velocity.
    (D) maintain a constant angular momentum.
    (E) maintain a state of rotational equilibrium.

45) A spinning star begins to collapse under its own gravitational pull. As it becomes smaller,
   (A) its angular velocity decreases.
   (B) its angular momentum increases.
   (C) its angular velocity remains constant.
   (D) its angular momentum remains constant.
   (E) both its angular momentum and its angular velocity remain constant.

Questions 46 through 50 pertain to the grindstone described below:

A grindstone of radius 2.0 m rotates about a fixed axis as shown at a constant angular speed of 5.0 rads/s.

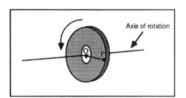

46) What is the tangential speed of a point on the rim of the grind stone?
   (A) 2.5 m/s   (C) 10.0 m/s   (E) zero
   (B) 5.0 m/s   (D) 5.0 m/s

47) What is the magnitude of the tangential acceleration of a point on the rim of the grindstone:
   (A) 2.5 m/s^2 (C) 10.0 m/s^2 (E) zero
   (B) 5.0 m/s^2 (D) 50.0 m/s^2

48) What is the magnitude of the centripetal acceleration of a point
on the rim of the grindstone:
(A) 2.5 m/s²   (C) 10.0 m/s²   (E) zero
(B) 5.0 m/s²   (D) 50.0 m/s²

For questions 49 and 50 consider the following statement concerning the same grindstone:

Suppose that the grindstone is stopped. Then, starting from rest. it is given an angular acceleration of 3.0 rad/s²

49) What is the angular displacement of the line OP (and hence the
grindstone) after 4.0 s?
(A) 6.0 rad   (C) 24.0 rad   (E) none of these
(B) 12.0 rad   (D) 48.0 rad

50) What is the angular speed of the grindstone after 4.0s?
(A) 6.0 rad   (C) 24.0 rad   (E) none of these
(B) 12.0 rad   (D) 48.0 rad

51) If the efficiency of a fixed pulley were 100%, the force required to lift a
block off the ground would be:
A) less than using an incline plane.
B) greater than using an incline plane.
C) equal to the force of the incline plane.
D) none of the above.

52) What is the mechanical advantage of a wheelbarrow if the load distance is
.5m from the fulcrum and the effort distance is 1.5m from the fulcrum?
A) .33
B) .3
C) .75
D) none of these

53) How much work is done by an elephant who is moving a circus tent 20m with a pulling force of 200N?
   A) 40000J
   B) 10J
   C) .1J
   D) none of these

54) When you turn a screw, the more times it is turned the greater the_____ will be.
   A) effort force
   B) afford load
   C) mechanical advantage
   D) all will be greater

55) If the mechanical advantage of a machine is two (2), then:
   A) the machine works twice as well as it's user.
   B) using the machine multiplies the resistance force by two.
   C) using the machine multiplies the effort of it's user by two.
   D) the machine cuts the amount of work to be done in half.

Questions 56 - 60 are True (T) or False (F):

56) Levers can increase effort force.

57) If the force being applied is 7N and the area is 14m Squared, then the pressure would be 2 pascals.

58) A grooved wheel with a rope or chain running through the groove is a compound machine.

59) Roller skates would be an example of a third class lever.

60) The rate at which work is done is called efficiency.

61) Two uncharged conducting spheres are suspended by nylon threads and touch each other. With a positively charged rod head near sphere 1, the two spheres are separated. How will the spheres be charged, if at all?

	Sphere 1	Sphere 2
(A)	0	+
(B)	-	+
(C)	0	0
(D)	-	0
(E)	+	-

62) Which statement best explains why tiny bits of paper are attracted to a charged rubber rod?
   (A) Paper is naturally a positive material.
   (B) Paper is naturally a negative material.
   (C) The paper becomes polarized by induction.
   (D) The paper acquires a net positive charge by induction.
   (E) The paper acquires a net negative charge by induction.

63) Two charged spheres are separated by a distance a. Which combination of charges on the two spheres will yield the greatest repulsive force?
   (A) 2q and -2q   (C) -3q and -2q   (E) +6q and -2q
   (B) +2q and +2q   (D) -3q and +2q

64) Which statement concerning a *conductor* in electrostatic equilibrium is *not* true?

(A) The electric field is zero in the interior of the conductor.

(B) The charge on the conductor is entirely on its outer surface.

(C) The electric field at the surface of the conductor is perpendicular to the surface.

(D) The electrostatic potential is non-zero throughout interior of the conductor.

65) Two particles of equal mass carry different charges of -q and +2q respectively.

They are shot along the positive x axis into a uniform electric field that points in the positive y direction.

Which will be the resultant paths for these particles?

(A) path 1 for -q and path 3 for +2q

(B) path 1 for +2q and path 3 for -q

(C) Path 2 for -q and path 3 for +2q

(D) Path 2 for +2q and path 4 for -q

(E) Path 2 for +2q and path 3 for -q

66) Which statement is true concerning the work done by an external agent in moving an electron at constant speed between two points in an electrostatic field?

(A) It is always zero.

(B) It is always positive.

(C) It is always negative.

(D) It depends on the total distance covered.

(E) It depends on the displacement of the electron.

67)   Which physical quantity is not correctly paired with its SI unit?

	Quantity	SI Unit
(A)	electric field	V / m
(B)	self-inductance	V - s / A
(C)	electric potential	Joule
(D)	magnetic field	Wb/m2
(E)	magnetic flux	Wb

68)   Which is true concerning the strength of the electric field between two oppositely charged parallel plates?
(A) It is zero midway between the plates.
(B) It is a maximum midway between the plates.
(C) It is a maximum near the positively charged plate.
(D) It is a maximum near the negatively charged plate.
(E) It is constant between the plates except near the edges.

Questions 69 and 70 pertain to the statement and diagram below:

The figure at the right represents a uniform electric field with magnitude 10^4 N/C that is directed toward the top of the page.

P and Q are points within the field and are separated by 0.1m

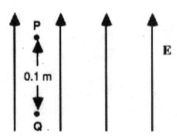

69) What force will be experienced by a $+20\mu C$ point charge placed at P?

   (A) 0.2 N directed toward to top of the page.

   (B) 0.2 N directed toward the bottom of the page.

   (C) 2×10^5 N directed toward the top of the page.

   (D) 2×10^8 N directed toward the top of the page.

   (E) 2×10^8 N directed toward the bottom of the page.

70) How much work is required for an external agent to move a charge of $-5uC$ from point P to point Q?

   (A) 0.01 J   (C) 0.2J   (E) none of these

   (B) 0.005J   (D) 5.0J

71) The *kilowatt hour* is a unit of

   (A) force   (D) electric field strength

   (B) energy   (E) electromagnetic induction

   (C) electrical power

Questions 72 through 74 pertain to the statement below:

Three parallel plate capacitors, each having a capacitance of 1.0 μF are connected in parallel.

72) What is the equivalent capacitance of this parallel combination?

   (A) 0.33 μF   (C) 1.0 μF   (E) 6.0d μF

   (B) 0.55 μF   (D) 3.0 μF

73) If a potential difference of 300 V is applied to the parallel combination, what would be the charge *on each* capacitor?

   (A) $1.0 \times 10^{-4}C$ (C) $9.0 \times 10^{-4}C$ (E) 9.0×10^8C

   (B) $3.0 \times 10^{-4}C$ (D) 3.0×10^8C

74) If a dielectric with constant κ=3 were added to each capacitor, what would the capacitance of each capacitor be?

(A) 0.33 uF   (C) 3.0 uF   (E) none of these
(B) 1.0 uF   (D) 6.0 uF

Questions 75 through 77 pertain to the situation described below:

Two charges of opposite sign and equal magnitude (Q =10 μC) are held 2 m apart as shown in the figure at the right.

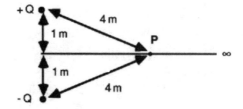

75) Determine the magnitude of the electric field at the point P.

(A) 2.8 x 10^{-3} N/C   (C) 2.8 x 10^2 NC   (E) zero
(B) 4.5 x 10^{-3} N/C   (D) 5.6 x 10^2 NC

76) Determine the electric potential at the point P.

(A) 1.1 x 10^{-3}V   (C) 4.5 x 10^{-3}V   (E) zero
(B) 2.2 x 10^{-3}V   (D) 9.0 x 10^{-3}V

77) How much work is required to move a 1μC charge from infinity to the point P?

(A) 1.1 x 10^{-3}J   (C) 4.5 x 10^{-3}J   (E) zero
(B) 2.2 x 10^{-3}J   (D) 9.0 x 10^{-3}J

Questions 78 and 79 pertain to the statement and diagram below:

Three resistors are wired as shown in the figure at the right.

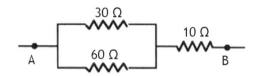

78.) What is the equivalent resistance between points A and B?
(A) 10Ω (C) 30Ω (E) 100Ω
(B) 20Ω (D) 50Ω

79) The potential drop between points A and B is 30 V. What is the potential drop across the 10Ω resistor?
(A) 10V   (C) 30V   (E) 100V
(B) 20V   (D) 50V

80) Which combination of units is equivalent to 1Ω?

(A) V/C   (C) J/s   (E) W/A
(B) A/J   (D) J s/C^2

Questions 81 through 83 pertain to the situation described below:

The figure at the right shows a simple RC circuit.

The capacitor is initially charged and just after the switch is closed, the charge on the capacitor is 30 μC.

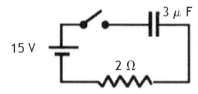

81) What is the potential drop across the resistor just after the switch is closed?

    (A) zero   (C) 10V   (E) none of these

    (B) 5V   (D) 37.5 W

82) At what rate is energy dissipated through the resistor in Joule heating *just after* the switch is closed?

    (A) 2.5W   (C) 12.5W   (E) 112.5 W

    (B) 1.5×10^{-4}J   (D) 37.5W

83) How much energy is stored in the capacitor just after the switch is closed?

    (A) zero   (C) 2.0×10^{-4}J   (E) none of these

    (B) 1.5×10^{-4}J   (D) 4.5×10^{-5}J

84) Which statement best explains why a constant magnetic field can do no work on a moving charged particle?

    (A) The magnetic field is conservative.

    (B) The magnetic field is a velocity dependent force.

    (C) The magnetic field is a vector and work is a scalar quantity.

    (D) The magnetic force is always perpendicular to the velocity of the particle.

    (E) The electric field associated with the particle cancels the effect of the magnetic field on the particle.

Questions 85and 86 pertain to the statement and figure below:

A long straight vertical wire traverses a magnetic field of magnitude 2T and with the direction shown in the diagram below. The length of the wire which is in the field is 0.06 m. When the switch is thrown, a current of 4 A flows through the wire from point P to point Q.

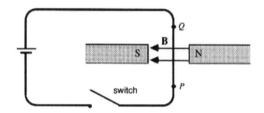

85) Which statement concerning the subsequent behavior of the wire is true?
    (A) It will be pushed to the left.
    (B) It will be pushed to the right.
    (C) It will remain in the position shown.
    (D) It will be pushed into the plane of the paper.
    (E) It will be pushed up out of the plane of the paper.

86) Determine the magnitude of the net force experienced by the wire.
    (A) 0.12N   (C) 0.48 N   (E) zero
    (B) 0.24 N   (D) 67.0 N

Questions 87 and 88 pertain to the two wire systems described below:

Two long straight wires carry currents in opposite directions as shown at the right.

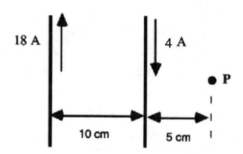

87) Determine the magnitude of the magnetic field at the point P.

(A) 2.4 x 10^{-5}T   (C) 7.2 x 10^{-5}T   (E) none of these

(B) 4.8 x 10^{-5}T   (D) 9.6 x 10^{-5}T

88) What is the direction of the magnetic field at the point P?

(A) to the left of the page   (D) into the plane of the page

(B) to the right of the page   (E) out of the plane of the page

(C) toward the bottom of the page

89) A charged particle of mass m, charge +q moves with speed v in a circle of radius R in a uniform magnetic field of magnitude B directed into the page as shown. The magnitude of the field is suddenly increased to 2B while the speed of the particle is maintained at v.

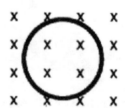

What is the radius of the particle's orbit after the field is doubled?

(A) R/2   (D) 4R

(B) R   (E) none of these

(C) 2 R

90) A proton traveling north enters a region which contains both a magnetic field and an electric field. The electric field lines point due west. It is observed that the proton continues to travel in a straight line due north. In which direction must the magnetic field lines point?

(A) up   (C) east   (E) south
(B) down   (D) west

Questions 91 and 92 pertain the situation described below:

The figure at the right shows a long straight wire in the plane of a rectangular conducting loop of resistance 2.0 Ω.

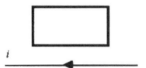

The wire carries a current in the direction shown in the figure.

91) Which entry in the table below correctly pairs the change in the system with the direction of the induced current around the conducting loop?

Change in the system	Direction of induced current around loop
(A) increased area of loop	no induced current
(B) pull loop toward top of page	clockwise
(C) decrease the magnitude of i	counterclockwise
(D) pull loop from left to right	clockwise
(E) maintain constant i in wire	counterclockwise

92. At what rate must the magnetic flux through the loop change with time if the induced current around the loop is 4A?
(A) 1 Wb/s   (C) 4 Wb/s   (E) none of these
(B) 2 Wb/s   (D) 8 Wb/s

93) The figure at the right shows a circular
conducting loop of resistance 3Ω that is
connected to a 5 V battery and a switch S.

Just after the switch s is closed, the
current through the loop changes
at a rate of 15 A/s. Determine the *self
inductance* of the coil.

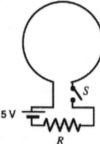

(A) 0.33 H   (D) 3.00 H
(B) 0.60 H   (E) 5.00 H
(C) 1.67 H

94.) A metal ring is moved to the left toward the south pole of a stationary
bar magnetic which is fixed in position as suggested in the figure
below.

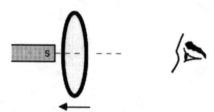

Which statement concerning this situation is true?
(A) Since the magnet is stationary, there will be no induced current
in the ring.
(B) As the ring is moved, an induced current will flow and appear
clockwise to the observer.
(C) As the ring is moved, an induced current will flow and appear
counterclockwise to the observer.
(D) As the ring is moved, there will be an induced magnetic field
around the right which appears to be *clockwise* to the
observer.
(E) As the ring is moved, there will be an induced magnetic field
around the right which appears to be *counterclockwise* to the
observer.

Questions 95 and 96 pertain to the situation described below:

An LC circuit is used to generate electromagnetic waves of frequency 100 Hz.

95) If the inductance of the circuit is 2.5H, what is the required value of the capacitance:

(A) 1F   (C) 1 x 10 $^{-3}$ F   (E) 100 μF

(B) 1uF   (D) 1x 10 $^{-12}$ ^{F}

96) At the instant when the charge on the capacitor is zero,

(A) the current in the circuit is zero

(B) the energy in the electric field is a maximum.

(C) the energy in the magnetic field is a maximum.

(D) the current through the inductor is *not* changing.

(E) the energy is equally shared between the electric and magnetic fields.

97) Which statement concerning electromagnetic waves is *not* true?

(A) They are longitudinal waves.

(B) They transfer energy through space.

(C) Their existence was predicted by Maxwell.

(D) They can propagate through a material substance.

(E) They do not require a physical medium for propagation.

Questions 98 and 99 pertain to the situation described below:

A beam of light which consists of a mixture of orange, yellow, and blue light strikes a prism as shown below. The prism is characterized by the indices of refraction for the various colors as indicated in the accompanying table

color	n
orange	1.37
yellow	1.44
blue	1.47

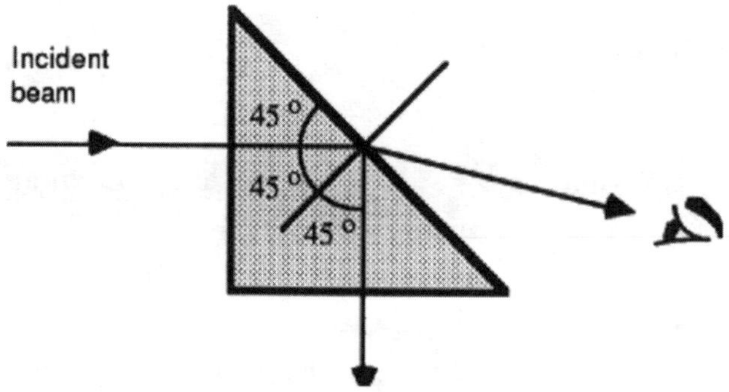

98) Which color(s), could in principle, be seen by an observer at A?
   (A) only blue light   (D) only blue and yellow light
   (B) only orange light   (E) only orange and yellow light
   (C) only yellow light

99) Which physical phenomenon is illustrated by the fact that the observer will not see all three colors of light?
   (A) dispersion   (D) interference
   (B) diffraction   (E) total internal reflection
   (C) Doppler effect

100) A physics student desires to create a beam of light that consists of parallel rays. How could this be accomplished?
(A) by placing a light bulb anywhere in front of a plane mirror
(B) by placing a light bulb at the focal point of a convex mirror
(C) by placing a light bulb at the center of curvature of a concave mirror
(D) by placing a light bulb at the center of curvature of a diverging lens
(E) by placing a light bulb at the focal point of a converging lens

101) An object is placed 15 cm from a converging lens of focal length 20 cm. how far from the object will the image be formed?
(A) 15cm   (C) 45cm   (E) 75 cm
(B) 20cm   (D) 60cm

102) The figure below shows the path of a portion of a ray of light as it passes through three different materials. *The figure is drawn to scale.*

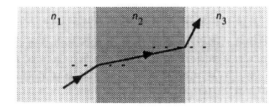

What can be concluded concerning the refractive indices of these three materials?

(A) n1 < nc <n3
(B) n1 > nc >n3
(C) n3 < n1 <n2
(D) n2 < n1 < n3
(E) No conclusion can be drawn without knowing

103) Which statement best explains why interference patterns are not usually observed for light from two ordinary light bulbs?
(A) Diffraction effects predominate.
(B) The two sources are out of phase.
(C) The two sources are not coherent.
(D) The interference patterns are too small to observe.
(E) The light from ordinary light bulbs is not polarized.

104) Two glass plates, each with index of refraction 1.55, are separated by a small distance D. The space between them is filled with water (n = 1.33).

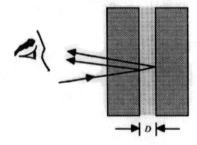

For which condition will the reflected light appear green? The wavelength of green light is 460 nm in vacuum.

(A) $D = \left[\dfrac{460 \text{ nm}}{2} \right]$ (D) $2D = \left[\dfrac{1}{2} \ \dfrac{460 \text{ nm}}{1.33} \right]$

(B) $2D = \left[\dfrac{460 \text{nm}}{1.33} \right]$ (E) $2D = \left[\dfrac{1}{2} \ \dfrac{460 \text{ nm}}{1.55} \right]$

(C) $2D = \left[\dfrac{460 \text{ nm}}{1.55} \right]$

Questions 105 through 108 pertain to the situation described below:

The figure below shows the interference pattern obtained in a double slit experiment with light of wavelength 600nm. The distance between the slits and the screen is close to 1m.

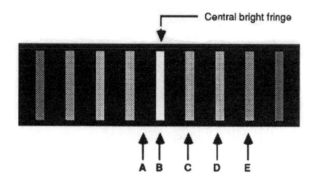

105) Which fringe is the *Third order maximum?*
   (A) A   (C) C   (E) E
   (B) B   (D) D

106) The angle that locates fringe A on the screen is 0.75°. Determine the slit separation d.
   (A) 400 nm   (C) 0.046 mm   (E) none of these
   (B) 0.023 mm   (D) 0.092 mm

107) Which fringe could be 1.0013746 m from one slit and 1.0013734 m from the other slit?
   (A) A   (C) C   (E) indeterminate from the information given
   (B) B   (D) D

108) Which would occur if the wavelength of the light were increased?
   (A) The fringes would become brighter.
   (B) More bright fringes would appear on the screen.
   (C) The central bright fringe would change position.
   (D) The distance between the dark fringes would decrease.
   (E) The angle that locates any bright fringe would increase.

109) The results of special relativity indicate that
   (A) Newtonian mechanics is an incorrect theory.
   (B) Moving clocks run fast compared to when they are at rest.
   (C) Moving objects appear to be longer than when they are at rest.
   (D) Newtonian mechanics is a valid approximation at low speeds ($v \ll c$).
   (E) The laws of electromagnetism are invalid for any observers that are in motion.

110) Which of the following characteristics of light requires that light is described in terms of particles or photons?
   (A) the photoelectric effect and Young's experiement
   (B) polarization experiments and Young's experiment
   (C) the diffraction of light and polarization experiments
   (D) light diffraction and the radiation spectrum from hot objects
   (E) the photoelectric effect and the radiation spectrum from hot objects

111) Science is related to technology as
   (A) potential energy is to kinetic energy
   (B) density is to specific gravity
   (C) hypothesis is to scientific law
   (D) research is to development

112) "The ringing sound of a bell cannot be heard in a vacuum."
Which subdivision of physics would be studied?
A) quantum mechanics and heat   C) electricity and magnetism
B) acoustics   D) nuclear and particle physics

113) A pendulum experiment yields the following values for acceleration due to gravity:

Trial	1	2	3	4	5
$g(m/s^2)$	9.350	9.345	9.350	9.350	9.348

Which statement best describes the results?
A) Accuracy is good; Precision is good.
B) Accuracy is good; Precision is poor.
C) Accuracy is poor; Precision is good.
D) Accuracy is poor; Precision is poor.

114) A person standing in an elevator which goes up with constant upward acceleration exerts a push on the floor of the elevator whose value
A) is always equal to his weight.
B) is always greater than his weight.
C) is always less than his weight.
D) is greater than his weight only when his acceleration is greater than g.

115) Two small masses, when 10 cm apart, attract each other with a force of F newtons. When 5 cm apart, these masses will attract each other with a force, in Newton's, of

A) F/2   C) F/4
B) 4F   D) 5F

The following graph refers to questions 116 - 119.

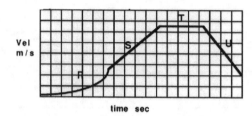

116) Which portion of the graph is Newton's 1st law being
      demonstrated?
      A) R   B) S   C) T   D) U

117) Which portion of the graph is the net force zero?
      A) R   B) S   C) T   .)U

118) Which portion of the graph illustrated deceleration?
      A) R   B) S   C) T   D) U

119) Which portion(s) of the graph is a variable force being applied?
      A) R   B) S   C) T   D) U

120) Two forces act on an object. The magnitude of their resultant is
     least when the angle between the forces is
     A) 0°   B) 45°   C) 90°   D) 180°

121) A girl in a train heading north at 40 m/s throws a ball out of the
     window at a speed of 30 m/s in an eastward direction. What is the
     velocity of the ball?
     A) 50 m/s; 37° from north   B) 70 m/s; 53° from east
     C) 50 m/s; 53° from north   D) 30 m/s; from east

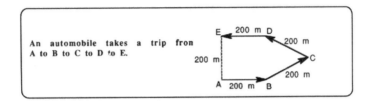

Study the information above; then complete sttements 122-123

An automobile takes a trip from A to B to C to D to E.

122) The total distance the automobile travels is
   A) 0 m   B) 200 m   C) 800 m   D) 1000 m

123. The displacement of the automobile from its starting point A is
   A) 0 m   B) 800 m   C) 200 m   D) 1000 m

124) A handball is tossed vertically upward with a velocity of 19.6 m/s.
   How high will it rise?
   A) 1.0 m   B) 9.80 m   C) 19.6 m   D) 30.0 m

125) A car going around a certain curve at a speed of 24.6 m/s has a
   centripetal force acting on it of 1000 N. If the speed of the car is
   doubled, the centripctal force

   A) is quadrupled   C) is reduced by one-half
   B) is doubled   D) is reduced by one-fourth

126) If the speed of an object is tripled, its kinetic energy is _____times
   that of its original speed.
   A) 1/9   B) 1/3   C) 3   D) 9

For questions 127-128 refer to:

A person having a mass of 60 kg exerts a horizontal force of 200 N in pushing a 90-kg object a distance of 6 meters along a horizontal floor. He does this at constant velocity in 3 seconds.

127) The work done by this person, in joules is
      A) 540   B) 1080   C) 1200   D) 3600

128) The force of friction is
      A) exactly 60 N   C) between 60 N and 90 N
      B) exactly 200 N   D) greater than 200 N

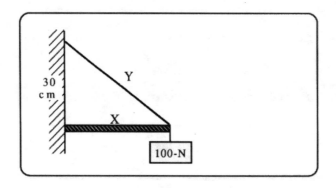

129) An object weighing 100 newtons is suspended from one end of a horizontal rod X. The other end of the rod rests against a vertical wall. The weight of the rod is negligible. The system is kept in equilibrium by rope Y, one end of which is attached to the same end of the rod as the weight. The other end of the rope is attached to a point on the wall 30 cm above the rod. The rod is 40 cm long. the tension in rope Y is
      A) 70N   B) 90N   C) 100N   D) 167 N

130) Two metal blocks seem to lose the same weight when completely submerged in liquid. According to Archimedes; principle, the objects must have the same
A) weight in air   C) volume
B) weight in water   D) density

131) When a liquid is boiling
A) its temperature remains constant
B) the kinetic energy of its molecules increases
C) a dissolved solid lowers the boiling temperature
D) a dissolved gas increases the boiling temperature

132) The term Brownian movement refers to
A) irregular motions of small particles suspended in a fluid
B) convection currents in a liquid or a gas
C) the stretching of a body beyond its elastic limit
D) the sinking of mercury in capillary tubes

133) The unit which does not represent the same physical quantity as the others is the
A) BTU   C) calorie
B) horsepower   D) joule

Refer to the Following Graph to Answer Questions 134 - 136

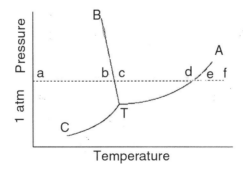

134) In the area BTC, water is

    A) solid   B) liquid   C) gas   D) vapor

135) The vapor pressure curve for water is curve

    A) TA   B) TB   C) TC   D) ATC

136) The heat required per unit mass for the phase change at point b-c
      is the

    A) heat of fusion.   C) specific heat

    B) thermal energy   D) heat of vaporization.

137) The two thin tubes which show most correctly the behavior of
      water are:

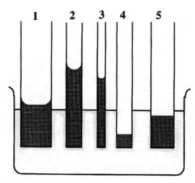

    A) 1 and 2   B) 3 and 4   C) 4 and 5   D) 1 and 4

138) If a man moves with a speed equal to 0.5 that of sound, away from a
      stationary organ producing a sound of frequency f, he would probably
      hear a sound of frequency

    A) 2.5f B) 1.5ff C) f D) less than f

139) If a vibrating body is to be in resonance with another body, it must

    A) be of the same materiel as the other body

    B) vibrate with the greatest possible amplitude

    C) have a natural frequency close to the natural frequency of the
       other body

    D) vibrate faster than usual

140) If a sound seems to be getting louder, which of the following is probably increasing?
A) intensity
B) frequency
C) wavelength
D) pitch

141) These waves are called square pulse waves. When Wave I is superimposed on Wave II they add to make the wave shown in

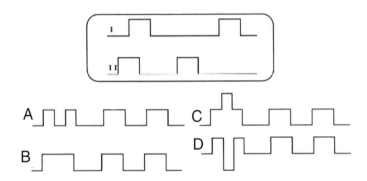

142) A stretched string produces a frequency of 1000Hz. If the same string is to produce a frequency twice as high, the tension of the string should be
A) doubled
B) quadrupled
C) reduced to 1/2 the original value
D) increased by a factor of $\sqrt{2}$

143) A small light source whose luminous intensity is 160 candela is located 2.0 meters above a horizontal table. The illumination of the table directly below the light source is, lumens/m²,
A) 40
B) 80
B) 320
D) 640

For questions 144 - 145 refer to:

A candle 6 inches long is placed upright front of a concave spherical mirror whose focal length is 10 cm. the distance of the candle from the mirror is 30cm

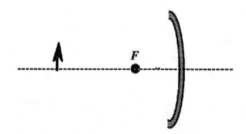

144) The radius of curvature of the mirror is
    A) 5cm   B) 10 cm   C) 15 cm   D) 20 cm

145) The image will be
    A) virtual and smaller than the candle
    B) virtual and larger than the candle
    C) real and smaller than the candle
    D) real and larger than the candle

146) The diagram represents wave fronts passing through a small
      opening in a barrier. This is an example of

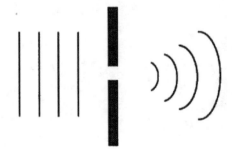

    A) reflection   B) refraction   C) polarization   D) diffraction

147) Two pulses approach each other in a spring, as shown.

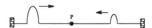

Which of the following diagrams best represents the appearance of the spring shortly after the pulses pass each other at point P?

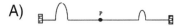

148) The speed of light in a certain transparent substance is two-fifths of its speed in air. The index of refraction of this substance is
A) 0.4   B) 1.4   C) 2.0   D) 2.5

149) The leaves of a negatively charged electroscope diverged more when a charged object was brought near the knob of the electro-scope. the object must have been
A) a conductor   C) negatively charged
B) an insulator   D) positively charged

150) Heating a magnet will
A) weaken it   C) strengthen it
B) have no effect   D) reverse its polarity

151) In the circuit shown, R_1 and R_2 are 30Ω and 60Ω respectively.

    I1 = 4 amp. The potential difference across R_2 is equal to

    A) 30 V   B) 60V   C) 120V   D) 240V

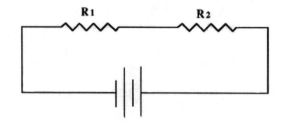

152) If a current-carrying wire runs directly over a magnetic compass, the needle of the compass will

    A) not be affected by the current

    B) point in a direction perpendicular to the wire

    C) point in a direction parallel to the wire

    D) tend to point to due north

153) When electric current in two parallel wires is flowing in the same direction, the wires tend to

    A) repel each other

    B) attract each other

    C) exert no force on each other

    D) twist at right angles to each other

154) A length of wire is coiled around an iron cylinder

    A) If current is made to flow in the wire, the iron becomes a magnet

    B) If the iron is a magnet, current is made to flow in the wire

    C) Both of the first two statements are true

    D) Both of the first two statements are false

155) An electron oscillating back and forth 1000 times each second will generate an electromagnetic frequency of

    A) 0 Hertz   C) 1000 Hertz

    B) 0.001 Hertz   D) 2000 Hertz

156) When a beta particle is emitted from the nucleus of an atom, the effect is to
   A) decrease the atomic number by 1
   B) decrease the mass number by 1
   C) increase the atomic number by 1
   D) increase the mass number by 1

157) Gamma rays consist of
   A) helium nuclei
   B) hydrogen nuclei
   C) high speed neutrinos
   D) radiation similar to X-rays

158) Neutrons penetrate matter readily chiefly because they
   A) occupy no more than one-tenth of the volume of electrons
   B) occupy no more than one-tenth of the volume of protons
   C) are electrically neutral
   D) are needlelike in shape

159) A photon whose energy is Ep joules strikes a photosensitive surface whose work function is W joules. The maximum energy of the ejected photoelectron is equal to
   A) Ep
   B) Ep + W
   C) Ep - W, only when Ep > W
   D) W - Ep, only when W > Ep

160) Consider the nuclear reaction:

$$_{1}^{2}H + _{1}^{3}H \Rightarrow _{2}^{4}He + _{0}^{1}n$$

This reaction is primarily an example of
   A) fission
   B) fusion
   C) alpha decay
   D) ionization

161) The cell structure which contains the chromosomes is the
  A) nucleus   C) mitochondrion
  B) cell wall   D) lysosome

162) Which of these organelles is surrounded by a membrane?
  A) vacuole   .   C) nucleus
  B) mitochondrion   D) all of the above

163) The cell theory for animals was formulated by
  A) Matthias Schleiden   C) Theodor Schwann
  B) Rudolf Virchow   D) Robert Brown

164) Which of the following is an example of a prokaryotic cell?
  A) liver cell   C) bacterial cell
  B) onion epidermis cell   D) mushroom cell

165) The cellular structures which release energy to support other cell activities are
  A) plastids   C) cell walls
  B) nucleoli   D) mitochondria

166) An organelle which contains protein-digesting enzymes is the
  A) chloroplast   C) vacuole
  B) lysosome   D) Golgi body

167) Which of the following is an example of a eukaryote?
  A. moss   C) human being
  B. both A and B   D) neither a nor b

168) Which structure is found only in bacterial cells?
  A) cell wall   C) cell membrane
  B) mitochondrion   D) nucleus

169) If a mitochondrion was defective, what aspect of the cell would be affected?
  A) reproduction   C) energy production
  B) protein synthesis   D) transport of secretions

170) The helical structure of DNA was discovered by
  A) Leeuwenhoek and Brown   C) Virchow and Malpighi
  B) Schleiden and Schwann   D) Watson and Crick

171) Which of these structures would contain protein-synthesizing enzymes?
   A) mitochondrion   C) lysosome
   B) ribosome   D) plastid

172) A strong salt solution will cause an onion cell to collapse because the solution is
   A) hypotonic   C) isotonic
   B) hypertonic   D) turgid

173) An egg without its shell would do what if put into a beaker of distilled water?
   A) collapse   C) swell
   B) stay the same   D) grow a shell

174) When the concentration of solutions on either side of a membrane is the same, the system is said to have reached
   A) equilibrium   C) plasmolysis
   B) condusion   D) cytolysis

175) An egg without its shell would do what if put into a strong sugar(concentrated) solution?
   A) collapse   C. swell
   B) stay the same   D) turn black

176) Osmosis is the diffusion of
   A) oxygen   C) matter
   B) water   D) vinegar

177) The term tissue fits which of the following?
   A) brain   C) blood
   B) endoplasmic reticulum   D) stomach

178) Diffusion is the random movement of
   A) cells   C) molecules
   B) organisms   D) cell membranes

179) The cell membrane lets only some things in and out. This makes it
   A) permeable   C) selectively permeable
   B) diffusion   D) osmosis

180) The cells you used to study plasmolysis were
   A) Elodea   C) red onion
   B) tomato   D) cork

181) Hydrogen released from glucose goes through the electron transport system as part of what process?
   A) photosynthesis   C) fermentation
   B) Krebs cycle   D) respiration

182) Which of the following is oxidized in the cells of many organisms to produce energy?
   A) NADP   C) glucose
   B) ATP   D) alcohol

183) Which of the following is part of the anaerobic stage of respiration?
   A) fermentation   C) photosynthesis
   B) glycolysis   D. light phase

184) Which of the following is a hydrogen acceptor?
   A) ADP   C) ATP
   B) NADP   D) glucose

185) An energy-releasing process of microbes which is used in the manufacture of bread and wine is
   A. lactic acid fermentation   C. alcoholic fermentation
   B. photosynthesis   D. respiration

186) During glycolysis, how many molecules of ATP are generated from one molecule of glucose?
   A) 1   C) 2
   B) 18   D) 36

187) Which of these processes is aerobic?
   A) Krebs Cycle   C) electron transport system
   B) Calvin cycle   D) glycolysis

188) Which of the following is not part of cellular respiration?
  A) glycolysis   C) Calvin cycle
  B) electron transport system D) Krebs cycle

189) The production of alcohol as by-products of energy release occurs in
  A) fermentation   C) photosynthesis
  B) glycolysis   D) the Calvin cycle

190) The following equation represents the summary reaction for what process?

$$C_6H_{12}O_6 + 6O_2 = 6CO_2 + 6H_2O + energy$$

  A) photosynthesis   C) cellular respiration
  B) alcoholic fermentation   D) lactic acid fermentation

191) The reactions of respiration take place in the
  A) cytoplasm and mitochondria C) mitochondria only
  B) cytoplasm only   D) chloroplast

192) Pyruvic acid is made during the reactions of
  A) glycolysis   C) Krebs cycle
  B) photosynthesis   D) Calvin cycle

193) The process of assembling protein molecules is called
  A) replication   C) transcription
  B) translation   D) bondin34.

194) Where does the production of RNA take place?
  A) in the nucleus   C) in the ribosomes
  B) in the cytoplasm   D) in the proteins

195) In DNA, thymine always bonds with
  A) cytosine   C) guanine
  B) uracil   D) adenine36.

196) A specific group of 196. three sequential bases of mRNA is called
  A) sugar   C) amino acid
  B) cluster   D) codon

197) Where does the process of translation occur?
      A) in the nucleus   C) at the ribosomes
      B) in the cytoplasm   D) in the Golgi apparatus

198) Which of the following is NOT a characteristic of RNA?
      A) uradil is present   C) single-stranded
      B) made by transcription   D) deoxyribose sugar is
                                        present

199) What must occur before DNA can replicate?
      A) RNA must be synthesized   C) the strands of DNA must
                                        separate
      B) RNA polymerase must bind   D) the genetic code must be
                                        changed

200) One of the main functions of DNA is to
      A) produce bases   C) break apart RNA
      B) make hydrogen bonds   D) store hereditary information

201) Proteins are composed of
      A) nucleotides   C) nitrogen bases
      B) deoxyribose   D) amino acids

202) If one strand of DNA reads CCCGAT, the complementary
      sequence must be
      A) CTTAGC   C) GGGCTA
      B) AAATCGD   D) GGGCTT

203) If one strand of DNA reads TAACGT, the sequence of mRNA
      produced from it would read
      A) ATTGCA   C) ATTGCC
      B) AUUGCA   D) UTTGCU

204) A trait that occurs in three individuals out of a total of four
      individuals occurs with a probability of
      A) 1/4   C) 2/4
      B) 3/4   D) 4/4

205) Mendel obtained his PURE F1 generation by allowing the plants to
A) self-pollinate   C) cross-pollinate
B) assort independently   D) segregate

206) The transmission of traits from parent to offspring is called
A) dominance   C) heredity
B) segregation   D) independent assortment

207) Organisms that have two identical genes for a certain trait are said to be _____ for that trait.
A) haploid   C) homozygous
B) heterozygous   D) diploid

208) A segment of DNA on a chromosome that controls a particular hereditary trait is called a(n)
A) gene   C) nucleus
B) allele   D) phenotype

209) Curly hair is dominant over straight and black hair is dominant over brown. What would be the genotype of a parent who is heterozygous for curly hair and homozygous for brown hair?
A) Ccbb   C) ccbb
B) CCBb   D) ccBb

210) Pure red flowers cross with pure yellow flowers, and all of the offspring are orange. This cross is an example of
A) self-pollination   C) segregation
B) independent assortment D) codominance

211) Upper- and lowercase letters are used to represent
A) alleles   C) chromosomes
B) phenotypes   D) probability

In sheep, white wool is dominant over black wool. A heterozygous sheep is crossed with a black sheep.

212) What are the genotypes of the parents?
A) Wb and bb   C) WW and ww
B) Ww and ww   D) Bb and bb

213) Which of the following is not a probable genotype of the offspring?

A) WW

C) Ww

B) ww

D) None of the above

214) What is the probability that the offspring will have white wool?

A) 0/4

C) 1/4

B) 2/4

D) 4/4

215) What is the probability that the offspring will have black wool?

A) 0/4

C) 1/4

B) 2/4

D) 3/4

216) In a dihybrid cross, how many squares are necessary for all probable offspring?

A) 4

C) 8

B) 12

D) 16

217) The mutation that results when a piece of a chromosome breaks off and is lost is called

A) a nondisjunction

C) a translocation

B) a deletion

D) an inversion

218) A mutation in sex cells is called a

A) point mutation

C) frameshift mutation

B) somatic cell mutation

D) germ cell mutation

219) An environmental factor that causes a mutation is called

A) an antigen

C) a monosomy

B) a trisomy

D) a mutagen

220) A mutation in which a piece of a chromosome breaks off and reattaches itself to a nonhomologous chromosome is called

A) a nondisjunction

C) a translocation

B) a deletion

D) an inversion

221) Which of the following is a type of gene mutation?

A) point mutation

C) shift mutation

B) inversion

D) mutagen

222) DNA stands for
   A) deribonucleic acid   C) deoxyribonucleic acid
   B) dynamic nucleic acids   D) denoxyacid

223) One of Mendels principles is the principle of
   A) heredity   C) segregation
   B) pollination   D) hybridization

224) Which of these factors would be likely to lower one's control
   (at rest) breathing rate?
   A) rebreathing exhaled air   C) exercise
   B) deep forced breaths   D) none of the preceding

225) The tube that carries urine from the kidney to the bladder is
   the called
   A) ureter   C) urethra
   B) uterus   D) renal vein

226) To test for sugar in the urine, you would use
   A) Biuret solution   C) Benedict solution
   B) glacial acetic acid   D) pH paper

227) The turbidity of urine is an expression of its
   A) color   C) pH
   B) cloudiness   D) all of the preceding

228) The air that leaves your lungs when the wind is knocked
   out of you is the
   A) tidal air   C) expiratory reserve volume
   B) inspiratory reserve volume   D) residual air

229) The order of air movement in the lungs is best described as
   A) bronchi to bronchioles to alveoli
   B) bronchi to alveoli to bronchioles
   C) bronchioles to bronchi to alveoli
   D) trachea to bronchi to alveoli

230) The smallest possible unit of a chemical compound is
    A) an electron
    B) a proton
    C) an atom
    D) a molecule

231) The direct change from the solid to gaseous state is referred to as
    A) melting
    B) boiling
    C) sublimation
    D) dissociatio

232) The formation of a chemical compound is invariably accompanied by
    A) absorption of heat
    B) release of heat
    C) either absorption or release of heat
    D) either absorption or release of kinetic energy

233) The reactions that are favored by light are called
    A) thermochemical reactions
    B) photochemical reactions
    C) exothermic reactions
    D) endothermic reactions

234) A decomposition of calcium carbonate into calcium oxide and CO_2
    $CaCO_3 = CaO + CO_2$ is an example of
    A) synthesis
    B) molecular rearrangement
    C) endothermic reaction
    D) exothermic reaction

235) A compound may be separated into its element by
    A) evaporation
    B) decomposition
    C) synthesis
    D) distillation

236) An unbalanced chemical equation is contrary to the law of
    A) gaseous volumes
    B) constant proportions
    C) conservation of mass
    D) mass action

237) The atoms of the isotopes of an element differ in the number of
    Λ) the electrons
    B) the protons
    C) the neutrons
    D) all the three fundamental particles

238) The atomic weight and atomic number of an element are W and N
      respectively. The number of neutrons in the atom of that element is
    A) W
    B) N
    C) N+W
    D) W-N

239) The atomic number of an element is 7. Its atom contains
    A) 7 electrons and 7 neutrons
    B) 7 protons and 7 electrons
    C) 7 neutrons
    D) 7 protons and 7 neutrons

240) Isotopes of an element have the same
    A) atomic weight
    B) atomic number
    C) number of neutrons
    D) number of nucleons

241) No two electrons in an atom can have all the four quantum numbers
      that are same. This principal is known as:
    A) exclusion principle
    B) uncertainty principle
    C) Hundís rule
    D) aufbau principle

242. Which one of the following statements is incorrect?
    A) electrons in motion display no properties that are identical to waves.
    B) an orbital can accommodate a maximum of two electrons
    C) *s*-orbitals have the shape of a sphere
    D) the energy of electrons in the various subshells increase in the following order: $s > p > d > zf$.

243. An element is best characterized by its:
    A) atomic weight
    B) atomic volume
    C) atomic charge
    D) chemical reactions

244. The configuration 1s22s12p3 represents:
    A) a nitrogen atom (ground state)
    B) a carbon atom (ground state)
    C) an excited carbon atom
    D) an excited nitrogen atom

245. Which one of the following does not consist of charged particles?
    A) alpha rays
    B) beta rays
    C) gamma rays
    D) none of the above

246. The particles emitted by radioactive elements are identical to electrons. Each electron ejected during beta emission comes from:
    A) the orbital electrons of the atom
    B) the nucleus of the atom
    C) a proton in the nucleus
    D) a neutron in the nucleus

247) Sublimation is an exothermic process.

    A) True   B) False

248) At the atmospheric pressure increases, so does the boiling point.

    A) True   B) False

249) As the polarity of a substance increases, so does its boiling point.

    A) True   B) False

250) The energy required to convert a solid to a liquid is refered to as the:

    A) Specific heat   C) Molar absorbtivity   E) Heat of vaporization

    B) Heat of sublimation   D) Heat of fusion

251) Which of the following represents a chemical change?

    A) Conversion of ice to steam   C) Combustion of natural gas

    B) Beer going flat   D) Leaves changing color in the fall

252) Convert 85 °F to Kelvin

    A) -243.6   B) 10.2   C) 29.4   D) 302.4

253). How many atoms in a sample of water that weighs 9.008 grams

    A)Not enough information   C) Avogadro's number

    B) 1/2 of Avogadro's number   D) 1.5 Avogadro's number

254) The maximum number of electrons that can occupy a 4d subshell is:

    A) 4   B) 6   C) 8   D) 10   E) varies

255) What is the most reasonable way for barium to achieve a noble gas configuration.

A) lose 1 electron C) share 6 electrons E) it already has a noble gas

B) lose 2 electrons D) gain 6 electrons configuration

256) If, during a chemical reaction, heat is given off, the reaction is:

A) exothermic C) isothermal E) evolutionary

B) endothermic D) isotonic

257) If 5 grams of hydrogen and 5 grams of oxygen are combined to form water, which substance would be considered the limiting reagent?

A) hydrogen C) water

B) oxygen D) none are limiting

258) You add 10 grams of a pure salt to water. After stirring the mixture for an hour and allowing it to stand, you observe a small amount of the salt at the bottom of the container. Under these conditions, you would expect the resulting solution to be:

A) unsaturated B) saturated C) supersaturated

259). A nitrogen gas sample is compressed to the point of liquification. This change is state is accompanied by which of the following changes.

A) Entropy and energy decrease

B) Entropy and energy increase

C) Entropy increases but energy decreases

D) Energy increases but entropy decreases

260) Which of the following is considered a weak acid?

A) nitric acid   C) sulfuric acid

B) hydrochloric acid   D) phosphoric acid

261) The ionization constant for a weak acid is referred to as it's:

A) Ka   B) Kb   C) Ksp   D) Kf

262) When the pressure on a gas increases, will the volume increase or decrease?

A) Increase
B) Decrease

263) Boyle's Law deals what quantities?

A) pressure/temperature   C) volume/temperature

B) pressure/volume   D) volume temperature/pressure

264) When the temperature of a gas decreases, does the volume increase or decrease?

A) Increase
B) Decrease

265) Charles' Law deals with what quantities?

A) pressure/temperature

B) pressure/volume

C) volume/temperature

D) volume/temperature/pressure

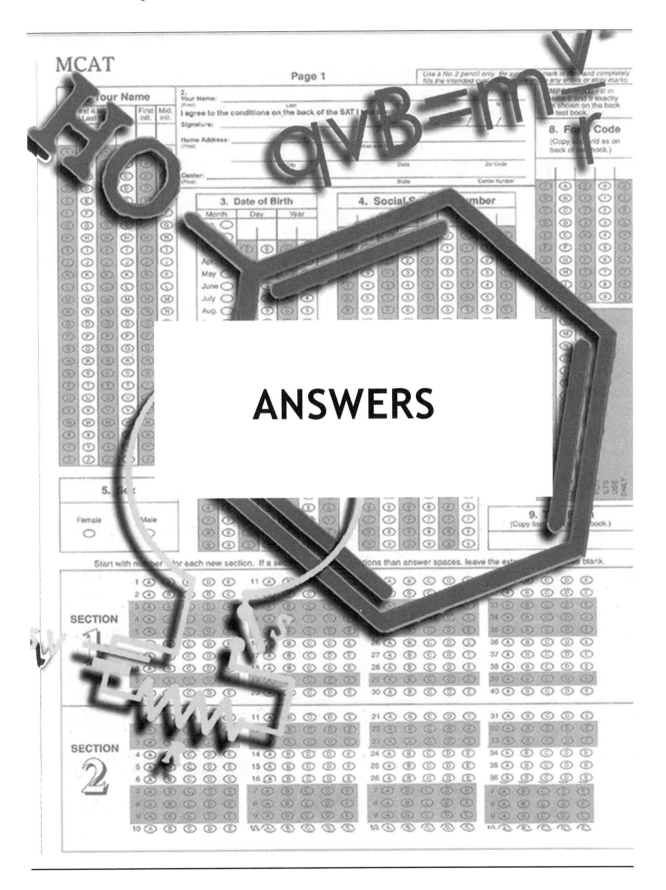

ANSWERS

PRACTICE QUESTION ANSWERS

1) E	34) B	67) C	100) E	133) B	166) B
2) B	35) C	68) E	101) C	134) A	167) B
3) B	36) B	69) A	102) C	135) C	168) A
4) C	37) C	70) B	103) C	136) A	169) C
5) D	38) C	71) B	104) B	137) A	170) D
6) A	39) E	72) D	105) E	138) D	171) B
7) C	40) A	73) B	106) B	139) C	172) B
8) D	41) A	74) C	107) D	140) A	173) C
9) C	42) B	75) A	108) E	141) C	174) A
10) D	43) B	76) E	109) D	142) B	175) A
11) C	44) C	77) E	110) E	143) A	176) B
12) B	45) D	78) C	111) D	144) D	177) C
13) E	46) C	79 A	112) B	145) C	178) C
14) E	47) E	80) D	113) C	146) D	179) C
15) E	48) D	81) B	114) B	147) B	180) A
16) A	49) C	82) C	115) B	148) D	181) B
17) E	50) B	83) B	116) C	149) C	182) B
18) A	51) B	84) D	117) C	150) A	183) A
19) B	52) D	85) D	118) D	151) D	184) B
20) B	53) A	86) C	119) A	152) B	185) C
21) A	54) D	87) A	120) D	153) B	186) C
22) C	55) C	88) D	121) A	154) A	187) A
23) D	56) T	89) A	122) C	155) C	188) A
24) A	57) F	90) B	123) C	156) C	189) A
25) A	58) F	91) C	124) C	157) D	190) C
26) A	59) T	92) D	125) A	158) C	191) A
27) C	60) F	93) A	126) D	159) C	192) A
28) B	61) B	94) C	127) C	160) B	193) A
29) C	62) C	95) B	128) B	161) A	194) A
30) D	63) C	96) C	129) D	162) D	195) D
31) D	64) D	97) A	130) D	163) C	196) D
32) C	65) B	98) B	131) A	164) C	197) C
33) E	66) E	99) A	132) A	165) D	198) D

199) C
200) D
201) D
202) C
203) B
204) B
205) A
206) C
207) C
208) A
209) A
210) D
211) A
212) B
213) A
214) B
215) B
216) D
217) B
218) D
219) D
220) C
221) A
222) C
223) C
224) C
225) A
226) C
227) B
228) A
229) A
230) C
231) C
232) C
233) B
234) D
235) B
236) C

237) C
238) D
239) B
240) B
241) A
242) A
243) A
244) A
245) C
246) D
247) B
248) A
249) A
250) D
251) C
252) D
253) B
254) D
255) B
256) A
257) B
258) B
259) D
260) D
261) A
262) B
263) B
264) B
265) C

QUESTIONS AND COMMENTS:
If you have suggestions for future card editions, please write or e-mail
suggestions to:
induspub@aol.com

FOR MORE INFORMATION ON
OTHER INDUS TITLES
VISIT OUR WEBSITE AT :
www.induspublishing.com

FUTURE TITLE
MCAT: The Answer Key 2
many more ready made index cards
with many more practice questions

MCAT RELATED TITLE

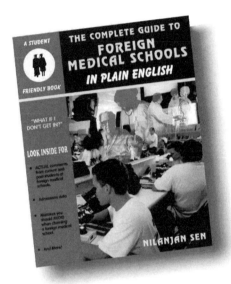